Essential Study Skills

Christine Ely BA MSc

*Senior Lecturer in Education, St Bartholomew School of Nursing and Midwifery,
City University, London, UK*

Ian Scott BSc PhD

*Senior Lecturer, Accreditation of Prior Experiental Learning,
St Bartholomew School of Nursing and Midwifery,
City University, London, UK*

Series Editor

Maggie Nicol BSc(Hons) MSc PGDipEd RGN

*Senior Lecturer, Clinical Skills and ILT Teaching Fellow,
St Bartholomew School of Nursing and Midwifery, City University, London, UK*

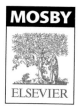

MOSBY

ELSEVIER

EDINBURGH LONDON NEW YORK OXFORD PHILADELPHIA ST LOUIS SYDNEY TORONTO 2007

MOSBY
ELSEVIER

The right of Christine Ely and Ian Scott to be identified as authors of this work has been asserted by them in accordance with the Copyright, Designs and Patents Act 1988

First published 2007

ISBN-13 978 0 7234 3371 2
ISBN-10 0 7234 3371 2

British Library Cataloguing in Publication Data
A catalogue record for this book is available from the British Library

Library of Congress Cataloging in Publication Data
A catalog record for this book is available from the Library of Congress

Notice
Neither the Publisher nor the authors assume any responsibility for any loss or injury and/or damage to persons or property arising out of or related to any use of the material contained in this book. It is the responsibility of the treating practitioner, relying on independent expertise and knowledge of the patient, to determine the best treatment and method of application for the patient.

The Publisher

10036770 8

Working together to grow libraries in developing countries

www.elsevier.com | www.bookaid.org | www.sabre.org

ELSEVIER   BOOK AID International   Sabre Foundation

your source for books, journals and multimedia in the health sciences
www.elsevierhealth.com

The
Publisher's
policy is to use
paper manufactured
from sustainable forests

Printed in China

Essential Study Skills

For Elsevier:

Senior Commissioning Editor: Ninette Premdas
Project Development Manager: Mairi McCubbin
Project Manager: Morven Dean
Design Direction: Judith Wright
Illustration Manager: Gillian Murray
Illustrations: Jonathan Haste

Contents

Preface

What we have to learn to do we learn by doing.
Aristotle 384–322 BC

Study skills are essential to nursing and the aim of this book is to provide you with an easy-to-use guide that will help you to develop the study skills necessary to your academic and professional life. If you have been working in or reading about the health service you cannot help but be impressed by the way in which nurses' roles have been changing and developing. How can we keep in touch with this constant change, so that nurses can adapt to the demands of their clients and community? This question affects a wide range of professionals and has been grappled with in recent times. The discussion has brought a new phrase and concept: 'lifelong learning'. Lifelong learning refers to the notion that individuals will engage with formal learning throughout their lives; what will be learned will be determined by the needs of the individual in response to challenges of their own and of society. Thus, education and continuing development will be an ever-present feature in the life of the nurse.

To cope with these changes and the volume of information around us, educational organisations have also been changing their approach to education. They are less concerned with ensuring that students can repeat large volumes of facts and figures than with helping students to discover how to learn for themselves. This book is designed to help you develop your skills in lifelong learning; to help you to understand yourself as a learner and to help you to become accomplished at knowing how to learn both theory and practical skills. We can learn through observing, listening, reading, doing and interacting with others. As well as helping you to become an efficient learner, this book will give you practical ideas and guidance that will help you succeed as a student.

Over a number of years we have helped, guided and watched a wide range of students develop and grow as competent learners and nurses. This has allowed us to gain an understanding of the skills and approaches to learning that will help students achieve their goals. Based on this experience and our observations with our students, we present in this book what we consider to be essential study skills. It aims to answer questions that students commonly ask about studying and learning at a university or higher education college. The chapters are illustrated throughout with examples showing how study skills are linked to nursing practice. Within each chapter additional sources of information that expand on particular issues are provided.

As well as helping to develop your skills we believe that this book will help you to generate the enthusiasm and motivation needed for study and that you will be able to see how to go about tackling new and exciting areas of study. It will supply direction; you may not know the most efficient way to approach your studies and need to be steered to finding appropriate information. We hope that by reading this book you will find support, discover the strategies that will work for you, and realise that there are many skills to being a lifelong learner and that most of us are not blessed with these skills at birth.

We start by introducing you to the institutions where you are likely to study nursing (universities and colleges of higher education). Practical advice is offered to help you adapt to a potentially demanding programme and set you up to succeed. The first chapters will help you gain an insight into what is involved in a pre-registration nursing course and provide ideas that will help you thrive during the first few weeks and adapt to the inevitable significant changes in your life. It is important to think about your learning during these early stages, as you will establish patterns and ways of working that are likely to remain with you throughout your time as a student nurse and beyond.

An important feature of these early stages is that you will need to manage your time so that you get the most from being a student. Time management is explored, and we look not only at how you can manage and plan your time effectively, but also how you can make the most of the time that you devote to your studies. We include areas such as self-motivation, how to remember more and how to identify your own preferred learning style.

As the book develops we explore the range of resources available to help you and how these resources can be used to benefit your studies. Advice is given on how to maximise physical resources, such as the library, as well as human resources, such as your tutors and lecturers. In Chapter 4, methods for searching databases and finding information are examined. We include here strategies for getting the most out of lectures and seminars, and how to read effectively. Approaches to making notes are outlined and the link between forming notes and how to develop understanding is also explored.

Chapters 5 and 6 are focused on presenting information. Knowing how to present information is an essential skill for those who wish to succeed at university and/or to work as a nurse. As a nurse you will need to be able to write notes and present your patient's case history. Chapter 5 looks at how to present work orally, how to improve basic writing skills and how to develop particular styles of writing. Chapter 6 develops the theme of presentation but is focussed on the types of assignment that you will be asked to complete at university or college. It examines how to manage and succeed at assignments such as essays and exams. These assessment techniques are essentially opportunities for you to present your ideas and thoughts on a particular topic.

Chapter 7 'How to learn practical nursing skills' explores techniques for learning clinical skills and what presentation skills are used when documenting nursing care and writing reports and patients' notes. In Chapter 8 'Learning from experience' we introduce the concept of reflection. Reflection is a technique whereby we look back, analyse and make sense of our experiences, thus helping us to learn from experience. Reflection is used extensively in nursing and other practice-based professions and is required in nurse education programmes to help you learn from experience, sometimes as part of assessments and also as a way of recording your experiences for future reference. In Chapter 8 we look at how reflective skills can be developed and how reflection is linked to professional development portfolios.

There is also a chapter on numeracy skills (Chapter 9). This has been included because using numbers is an important aspect of the day-to-day work of nurses, and nursing students frequently express a desire to be given more support in developing these skills. Because such skills are so important in nursing, many employers now test the numeracy skills of applicants for employment so it is as well to make sure that you are ready.

We hope that you enjoy using this book and find it helpful. We wish you every success in your future career.

Christine Ely

London, January 2006

Ian Scott

1

How to become a successful student nurse

Learning outcomes

This chapter is designed to help you:

- Understand what is involved when studying nursing at university
- Cope with the first few weeks of your course and adapt to student life
- Consider your health and safety as a student nurse
- Be aware of the financial issues involved when starting nursing
- Make the best use of student unions and professional bodies
- Keep motivated if things get tough.

INTRODUCTION

In the UK, nurse education for entry to the Nursing Register is now centred in universities. Like many other health-related professions that have also been incorporated into universities, this is to ensure that health care practitioners are given the appropriate preparation to meet the complex demands of twenty-first century health care. Rapid advances in health care mean that nurses are now required to a have a wider than ever range of knowledge and skills. Since the beginning of modern nursing in the nineteenth century, trainee nurses have studied their subject both in classrooms and in practice to ensure that they have the necessary knowledge and practical skills. This means that as a nursing student you will tend to work longer hours and have shorter holidays than other university students. This is because you are in effect working to obtain two qualifications at the same time: studying for a diploma or degree and your registration as a nurse. As with all subjects, learning about nursing is much easier if you are well organised and you can develop good study skills as you progress through the programme.

Although the idea of starting the new course will be exciting when you actually start, it may also seem somewhat daunting. However, things will be organised for you to help you settle in and get used to university life. First of all there is the challenge of starting your course and managing the first few weeks.

Coping with the first few weeks

In the transition to studying at university, you are likely to find that other students starting the programme with you may come from a variety of different educational and cultural backgrounds. Some students enter nursing straight from secondary school following GCSE or A levels and some from an access course, whereas others have completed NVQ qualifications while working in health care. Whatever you have done before; starting to study at university requires some adaptation. Getting used to large groups, meeting large numbers of staff and keeping track of names and faces can be exciting but also tiring. Make a careful note of the names of those who are managing your programme, so that you know who to contact if you have any queries. Departmental notice boards often have photographs of relevant individuals, or these may be displayed on websites if you are not sure who is who.

Notice boards and help points

Key information will be displayed at help points/help desks and notice boards. Make it a habit to check the relevant notice boards regularly as this is the means of communication that your tutors are most likely to use to convey information about timetables and tutorials. Changes to the printed timetable at some point are almost inevitable and these changes will usually be notified via the notice board or website. In addition, personal tutors are also likely to use the notice boards to arrange their first meeting with you.

Organising information

During the first few weeks you will, without doubt, be given large amounts of information verbally and in paper form or via your university's web pages. Although overwhelming at the beginning, it will all be important information that you will need during the course. File this information, so that you can find things later: a large ring binder file is probably best with dividers to sort it into sections. You will not usually need to carry this information around with you but will need to know exactly where to find what you need when working on assessments, etc., at home.

You will probably be given a number of handbooks and these should be kept in a safe place. Handbooks will cover things such as the university's rules and regulations, health and safety policies and usually information about course work and where to hand in your work. Try to focus on key information that you need now, and file other items in large ring binders or box files. Follow tutors' advice and read relevant parts which they point out as key information; alternatively, you may wish to skim read these initially and then look at them in more detail when you have settled into the course. The information that you need to focus on is your timetable, which you should examine carefully and check that you know exactly where you need to be and when. Get into the habit of preparing for lessons. Check out venues by ensuring you have relevant maps or directions and allow extra time to find new places; many universities have several different campuses.

Studying nursing at university

The most valuable study skill you can acquire as you adapt to life as a student is getting – and staying – organised. This may sound easy but finding time to study can be difficult at first. Modern lives tend to be busy and you need to decide how you will fit study into your life. Chapter 2 will give you an idea of what this might involve. Some important things to think of now are outlined below.

A university is a community of people whose goal is to study and research in order to learn about the world. Universities are made up of students, teachers (called tutors or lecturers) and researchers (who may also be lecturers). Research is the process by which much new information and knowledge is discovered and this key aspect of university life is essential to the development of a rapidly developing subject such as nursing. Your tutors and lecturers will be continuing their education to keep up to date and even studying for higher qualifications as well as conducting research. What this means, of course, is that they understand the demands of studying. Support staff, such as course administrators, are also there to help you as they keep everything running as smoothly as possible. As your course also includes clinical practice, the practice educators and mentors (see pp. 52, 53) will be an important part of the university community.

Transition to studying at university

As outlined in 'Coping with the first few weeks' above, students come from a variety of backgrounds. If you have previously been studying at sixth form or at a further education college doing an access course you will be used to the learning environment. This familiarity can help you make the transition to higher education.

If you have been working as a health care assistant or in other employment it may take a while to adjust to sitting and listening in class rather than being active 'doing things'. If you find this period of adaptation difficult, try talking to your personal tutor. However, be reassured that adapting to this sort of change can take a few weeks.

Clinical placements

You will not be in the university for all of the time because 50% of your time will be in a placement related to health care. Your role in the placement area will be as a student where the focus of your activity is learning rather than just getting work done. If you have previously been a health care assistant you will need to consciously make the transition to a learner. If you have no experience of working in health care then you will have to get used to hospital atmospheres, which can be daunting at first. However, be assured that you will quickly become familiar with placement areas. Remember your tutors and the staff in placement areas were all students once. Seeking help from your peers is a good study skill and more senior students will be in placement areas to help you adjust.

Preparing for placements

You will need to have a positive state of mind when going to a placement area. You must be physically fit as you will be actively involved in patient care and this means being on your feet for much of a shift. Nurses tend to have to do a lot of walking when at work and if you are used to being more sedentary for most of the day you must prepare yourself for this aspect of the placement experience. Although helpful, it is not necessary to go to the gym; do however, practise walking by incorporating one or two 20-minute brisk walks instead of bus rides or driving, into your daily routine.

You will need suitable clothing and footwear. It is usually suggested that you wear shoes that are black lace-ups which are flat healed and in a plain style. These may not be highly fashionable but your feet need to be protected if you are going to do a lot of walking. Trainers or sandals are not suitable. The course teacher or your handbook will often provide guidelines on appropriate footwear for placements. Your uniform should look smart and fit you in a way that allows freedom of movement; it is designed to be practical and allow safe moving and handling – it is not meant to be glamorous!

If you are to wear your own clothes on placement, ensure you follow any guidelines on appropriate dress. Always wear your name badge in accordance with university regulations. This will ensure that everyone knows you are a student and they can then be prepared to meet your educational needs. Looking like a nurse will help your confidence.

Learning to manage your time

A winning formula for success as a student nurse is learning how to manage your time well and using all the available resources to make studying easier. As you will spend half of your course in practice placements, time available for study will be precious and you need to make the best use of it. If you plan well, academic tasks such as reading and writing essays will not overwhelm you, and it will become a pleasure to learn rather than a chore. Managing the care of patients requires organisational skills and a sound knowledge of nursing, so effectively coping with your study will help in your development as a professional nurse. It will not just happen: you have to learn to plan your study activities to ensure your success. To plan your time effectively you need to:

- Find out approximately how many hours, on average, your course tutors advise you to study per week and then work out a weekly plan of how you are going to fit these hours into your schedule.
- As you undertake various study activities, keep a note of how long it actually takes; for example, to read and take notes from an article.
- Match your different study activities with the time available; for example, use quality time, such as when you are not likely to be interrupted and when you are feeling fresh, for reading which requires high levels of concentration. Leave sorting notes and filing items for times when you are not alone such as when you have to share the room with others watching television.
- After the first month or so make time to review how well your study plan is working and make further adjustments. This could be done with your personal tutor (see also Chapter 2).

Punctuality

Learning to be there or do things on time is essential. Ask family and friends for an evaluation of your punctuality and if they say you are often late then you need to change. If you arrive late for lectures or seminars you will feel flustered or you may not be allowed to enter the classroom as this is disruptive. You may have missed valuable information at the beginning of a session as most lecturers start by setting the scene and outlining the content. They may discuss important points about essays or exams and missing these can leave you floundering in the class, not quite sure what you are learning and why it is relevant. For practical sessions you may have missed essential health and safety instructions and your late entry would constitute a hazard.

Punctuality is very important in nursing practice and as most of your lecturers are nurses, they will expect you to be punctual. Arriving late is also disruptive to your fellow students, especially if they have to move to allow you to get to a seat. Some universities operate strict rules on lateness and will not allow students to enter more than 10 minutes after the lecture has started. Allow plenty of time to travel, especially at rush hour, and if you arrive early you can use any spare time in the library.

Attend every session

When you start the course there will be a lot of different subjects to cover. This will include biology, psychology, sociology, health promotion, ethical and legal issues, as well as nursing studies. Although some aspects of your studies may not seem relevant at first, you have to trust your lecturers. Some social science subjects, for instance, may seem abstract but your placement experiences will help you realise that patients can have complex social lives and problems that affect their health. Things will begin to make sense as you appreciate the wider social and political issues that have an impact on nursing. All the components of your programme are important and some aspects will only become relevant later in your studies.

Furthermore, because you are studying for a professional qualification, the university will need to ensure that you have attended a minimum number of sessions (usually over 80%) throughout the programme. There will usually be a system of registers to ensure that your attendance meets the minimum requirements.

The role of the lecturer and self-directed learning

From your time as a child at school you will be familiar with the concept of a teacher as one who instructs you and provides the knowledge you need to acquire. In adult education at university the lecturer is more likely to act as a facilitator of your learning. In other words, rather than just provide you with the knowledge, the lecturer will help you (facilitate you), either on your own or in a group, to seek out the knowledge for yourself. A significant amount of your learning will be directed by an awareness of your own learning needs. This is called self-directed learning and means that you are in control of how and when you learn.

> **Tip**
>
> Don't wait to be directed by others – be self-directed. Try to ask yourself questions before and after sessions and then try to find out information for yourself.

Self-directed learning can take a bit of getting used to as you may feel more comfortable with the idea of the teacher just instructing (as you did at school) rather than you, as an adult learner, having to find things out for yourself. However, this approach fosters independence in learning, which will prepare you for professional practice when you will be responsible for your own continuing education. Remember ... 'Learning can only be accomplished by the learner' (Rogers 1989: 40).

The advantage of learning through self-directed study is that you will learn at your own pace and you are more likely to understand and remember what you are learning. If you use self-directed study to prepare yourself for lectures by reading about the topic, you will find that the information is much easier to retain. In addition, you will be able to seek clarification from the lecturer about any aspects that you did not understand in your reading.

Changing roles: becoming a student

Your family may also need to make some adjustments when you become a student nurse. Changing roles in a family can impact on relationships: becoming a student can change the way you are perceived in the family. Having someone in the family studying a new subject can be very enriching; it can bring life and excitement, and your family will be very proud when you qualify. Try to keep your family involved with your progress, but be careful when discussing your placement experiences as this could cause distress and may even breach confidentiality. If you feel a need to talk about stressful events in school or placement, it may be best to discuss this with your personal tutor or placement mentor (see Chapter 3).

There is the potential for friction when you are studying to be a nurse, as your children or partner may feel you have less time for them and that you are less interested in their lives than before; your life may also have ceased to revolve around them. Be aware that your children and/or your partner may feel neglected and take steps to involve them in your studies. If they are aware of your progress and can see you nearing your goals, they can appreciate your success. They will be proud when you graduate.

Coming to a new country to study nursing can be immensely exciting but also hugely challenging. Not only will you have to adjust to a new course and be introduced to a new profession, but you will also have to get used to living in a different culture. If you have not undertaken any previous studying in English it is advisable to seek help with your written English early in the course. Help is usually available from the student support services and the Students Union (see p. 13).

Childcare issues

If you have to care for children or other dependants such as older relatives, you may be making big sacrifices in the short term in order to achieve your goal of becoming a nurse. If you have made the commitment to study to be a nurse, you will have to do it 100%. Although your university may be able to offer some flexibility, because of the nature of nursing it may be difficult for you to fit attending university campus and placement commitments with your home circumstances. Find out as much as possible before you start your programme about the demands that the course is likely to make on your time. You will need to arrange childcare that is compatible with shift patterns (Table 1.1). If you use a registered childminder in the UK you may be able to obtain funding to help with these costs. Seek advice from your student union or social services.

Placement shift patterns

All nursing programmes include placements in real care environments. In the UK you must spend 50% of your course in placement areas, and to be eligible to enter the Register for Nurses or Midwives you must have documentary proof of the exact number of hours you have completed in practice. As you will be expected to work as part of the care team, you must start when they start work and do the same shifts, which will usually be 7–8 hours long – sometimes even longer. Shifts will start either early in the morning (between 07.00 and 08.00) or early in the afternoon (around 13.00) and do not finish until after 21.00 or even later (Table 1.1). As a student you will be required to work some night shifts but this is not usually until the second or third year of your programme. It is a good idea to investigate what the travelling to and from placements would involve before you choose where to study. Many hospitals have restricted parking which may include a charge.

Table 1.1 Shift patterns

	Mon	Tues	Wed	Thurs	Fri	Sat	Sun
Week 1	07.30–15.30	13.00–21.00	07.30–15.30	13.00–21.00	07.30–15.30	Off	Off
Week 2	07.30–15.30	13.00–21.00	07.30–15.30	Off	Off	13.00–21.00	07.30–15.30
Week 3	07.30–15.30	13.00–21.00	07.30–15.30	13.00–21.00	07.30–15.30	Off	Off
Week 4	Off	Off	07.30–15.30	13.00–21.00	07.30–15.30	07.30–15.30	13.00–21.00

Preparing your study space

Planning to study includes making physical space at home to accommodate course work, your resources (e.g. books, files) and general information such as timetables. Plan where you are going to study, as you may need more space and some rearrangement of furniture may be required.

> **Tip**
>
> Avoid fatigue when studying – try to take a short break every 30 minutes as long periods of study, even with correct positioning and posture, can cause a strain on eyes and muscles.

Comfort is important in your study area as you need to feel that your study time is as pleasant and enjoyable an experience as possible.

You will need the following:

- Computer screen – make sure you adjust the angle and height so it is comfortable to work. The top of the screen should be roughly at eye level. Reduce the brightness if necessary.
- Keyboard – adjust the keyboard. You may find it better not to have this tilted if a high angle makes your wrists uncomfortable.
- Seating – adjust the height of the chair to the desk so that your lower arms are roughly horizontal to the desk. Your feet should be flat on the floor.
- Desk space – where you can leave papers and books out while doing assignments; a place where they will not be disturbed, especially by young children looking for paper to draw on!
- Book shelves – enough for at least 10 large books.
- Filing facility – either box files or a filing cabinet.
- Notice board – this is useful for timetables and duty rotas when on placements, and reminders, 'to-do' lists, etc.
- Internet access is usually available at the university but it will be a great help if you also have this at home. Searching for information on the internet can be done at any time of the day and therefore fits around other commitments. In addition, you

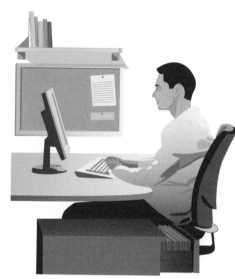

- **Computer screen** – make sure you adjust the angle and height so it is comfortable to work. The top of the screen should be roughly at eye level. Reduce the brightness if necessary.
- **Keyboard** – adjust the keyboard. You may find it better not to have this tilted if the angle makes your wrists uncomfortable.
- **Seating** – adjust the height of the chair to the desk so that your lower arms are roughly horizontal to the desk. Your feet should be flat on the floor.
- **Desk space** – where you can leave papers and books out while doing assignments; a place where they will not be disturbed, especially by young children looking for paper to draw on!
- **Book shelves** – enough for at least 10 large books.
- **Filing facility** – either box files or filing cabinet.
- **Notice board** – this is useful for timetables and duty rotas when on placements, and reminders, 'to-do' lists, etc.

Figure 1.1 Study space

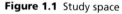

can renew library books, search the library catalogue and reserve books and access journals via the internet at most universities, so it is very helpful if you can arrange access at home. You may also find it helpful to keep in contact with colleagues and your personal tutor by email or electronic message boards.

- Computer access may need to be negotiated with others with whom you live, as they may be keen to play games or shop online just when you want to write an essay. Many universities require essays to be typed and, even if this is not a stipulation, using a word processor makes it much easier to revise your essay and send drafts (see Fig. 1.1) electronically to your tutor for comments.

Your health and safety as a student nurse

Health and safety is a key part of your academic and practical learning experiences. Nurses must have an understanding of health and safety legislation. In the UK this includes:

- The Health and Safety at Work Act 1974
- Control of Substances Hazardous to Health (COSHH) 2002 regulations
- Manual Handling Operations Regulations (MHOR) 1992.

The Health and Safety Executive website (www.hse.gov.uk/healthservices) can provide relevant information as to how these relate to working in a health care environment. As a student you must always familiarise yourself with emergency procedures as part of your health and safety induction (when you are shown around and told where safety information is in the area) whenever you commence a placement or go to a new environment for lectures.

As a qualified nurse you will be required to have regular training updates related to health and safety issues. Get into the habit of recording this information. At the commencement of your programme you should take responsibility for maintaining records of health and safety training in your portfolio (see Chapter 8) which will include fire, manual handling and first aid including cardiopulmonary resuscitation (CPR). It is essential that you attend these sessions and failure to do so may mean that you cannot go to your clinical placement.

> ### Tip
> Get into the habit of recording your attendance at all health and safety-related sessions in your portfolio.

Your physical and mental health

A medical assessment is normally required prior to starting placements as nursing is a physically demanding profession: you need to be fit both physically and mentally to study as a student nurse. Looking to the future, in order for you to register as a nurse you will need to provide a written declaration that you are in good health. Nursing can be a stressful occupation because you will encounter seriously ill and dying patients, which understandably may be upsetting. In addition, studying can be stressful. However, not all stress is bad as it can act as a motivator. To study effectively you need to develop effective coping mechanisms to manage stress, such as using physical exercise and getting support when needed.

Physical exercise is really beneficial. This does not have to be a sport or going to the gym if you are not keen on these; brisk walking for at least 20 minutes a day will be equally beneficial, as will activities such as dancing or relaxation classes. Try getting off the bus or train one stop early and having a brisk walk the rest of the way. If you have children and there is little time for these things, try joining your children when they go swimming or walking. If stressful events are affecting your studies, seek advice from your personal tutor, a member of the occupational health service or the student counselling service in the university. They are there to help keep you healthy. As a health professional you will be promoting the benefits of exercise.

A significant part of the nurse's role is to be a health educator. To have credibility in this area you must present a positive health image. You should appear physically fit and be able to carry out the duties expected of a nurse. You will need, for example, to be able to spend a considerable part of the day on your feet, so choosing the right footwear is important, as is the fit of your uniform which should be loose enough to allow a full range of movement (see 'Preparing for placements' above).

Care for your back when studying

Strain injuries can occur when studying. Ensure your computer area and seating are correctly adjusted to your physical needs (see 'Preparing your study space' above). You must also take care to avoid musculoskeletal injuries when carrying heavy books and folders. Try to study in the library rather than carry very heavy books home. Think about a case with wheels or a backpack rather than carrying bags, which might strain your back. Nurses belong to an occupational group that is particularly prone to back injuries, so remember to practise good handling techniques, not only in placement, but also in every activity in your daily life.

Personal safety

As a student nurse you need to think of your personal safety. Although the likelihood of an attack is small, you must be aware that you may be vulnerable both travelling to and from placements and university. Your university may provide written information about personal safety. Even if you feel you are pretty streetwise, you must learn how to avoid risks, particularly when travelling late at night. Take a careful note of all advice provided on security matters. The following personal safety strategies are based on advice from the Suzy Lamplugh Trust (www.suzylamplugh.org.uk):

- If your allocated placement is new to you, check it out in daylight before you commence the first shift.
- It is dangerous to travel around in your uniform and your university policy will probably not allow it; it is both unhygienic and invites inappropriate attention from some members of the public. People with criminal intent may assume that you have medicines in your bags.
- When travelling, keep valuables, including mobile phones, and laptops out of sight. Keep a copy of all the numbers on your mobile phone and do not carry address books in your handbag in case it gets stolen.
- Stay alert and aware of your surroundings – personal stereos and long mobile phone conversations can be a distraction when you are alone and you may not see someone approaching you.
- Avoid alleyways, underpasses and unlit car parks at night when alone.
- While you are on placement or in the university, the security services will endeavour to protect you and your property; however, as with all organisations where there is access for the public, there is always the potential for 'walk-in theft' so look after your valuables at all times. It is best to carry as few valuables as possible as there may not be any secure places to leave them.
- Protect your identity as a student by being careful with your placement documents, university ID and uniforms. If stolen, these forms of identity can provide the opportunity for criminals to impersonate you and then steal from patients or pretend to be a student to gain illegal employment.
- When approaching your home you should have keys ready so that you do not have to spend time looking in a bag, which would allow someone to approach without you noticing.
- Always be alert for people waiting outside nursing residencies and accommodation, and do not allow them access when you go in. If necessary, go away again and alert security services.
- If you live in your own home, review the security outside your door. Make sure there are no places where an intruder can hide such as tall bins or hedges. Ensure your doorway is well lit; a light that comes on as you walk towards it is helpful.
- Have an action plan in case of a security problem – people you can contact, such as neighbours or local shopkeepers.

Financial issues

Financial problems are known to be one of the reasons why some students do not complete their studies. It is very important that you think carefully about your resources at the start of your course. Just as you need to manage your time, you also need to manage your money. Some of your outgoings may be fixed costs (i.e. those you can do little to change such as rent or child care costs) but others such as your mobile phone bill can be reduced. Text messaging and email, for example, can be much more cost effective forms of communication.

Working out a budget, detailing your income and outgoings is essential; if you are relatively new to handling large sums of money you may want to consult someone who has had more experience. Good sources are your student union (see p. 13). Loans may seem an easy way out, but can be expensive in the long term. High rates of interest are charged to those without fixed assets. UK health care students in receipt of a bursary are currently not entitled to a government student loan but you may be eligible for state benefits or help with housing costs. Social Services or the local Citizens Advice Bureau should be able to provide more information.

Your bursary is administered through the Students' Grant Unit (not by your university) and you will need to contact the Unit directly if you have any problems concerning your bursary. Your university will give you the relevant telephone numbers or websites.

The Department of Health also provides a useful booklet of information on bursaries and this can be obtained from your university or college.

> ### Tip
> Seek help sooner rather than later if you are experiencing financial difficulties. Most organisations will try to help by reducing or deferring payments, but talk to them before these problems escalate.

There are also, often, hardship funds available through the university (see p. 13), which may be able to help if you have a financial problem. These funds can be applied for if you meet certain criteria and are able to supply evidence of financial difficulties. The student union will have advice officers who can give further information on accessing such funds and may also be able to give information on other sources of funding for students.

Part-time work

You might consider undertaking part-time work, possibly working as a health care assistant, to boost your income; however, this must not be at the expense of your study time. Undertaking too much part-time work may cause stress and tire you for classroom sessions. Students who miss classes are more likely to fail assessments. Working a few shifts as a health care assistant when you are on holiday or at weekends may be helpful as it can provide you with extra experience and more opportunities to practise the skills that you are learning. However, if you find yourself having to work increasingly long hours, you need to reassess your situation. Discuss this issue with your personal tutor.

The Student Union and professional bodies

Your university will provide information about its own student union, either on the website or in student handbooks. This organisation will provide advice on financial problems, housing and legal issues. You can also get more information with regard to concessions available to you (e.g. travel) as a student. The National Union of Students is a student-led organisation that campaigns for students' rights and welfare, and has special interest groups. More information can be found on their website, www.nusonline.co.uk

Student advisors

There may be times when you need help which is beyond the scope of your personal tutor. Universities provide staff for advice and guidance with regard to career choices and offer confidential counselling services. It is likely that you will be introduced to these services when you commence your programme and there should be further information in your student handbook or on the university website.

> **Tip**
>
> If you feel you have chosen the wrong branch of nursing you may be able to change at the end of your foundation year. Discuss this with those who coordinate the programmes so that you have all the information you need to make the right choice.

Professional bodies and health care unions

Professional bodies and the unions representing health care workers offer reduced rate membership for students and will provide support and advice for student nurses. They may also give access to a wide range of learning resources and other materials that relate to the nursing profession. You may benefit from contact with other student nurses through these bodies with whom you can share experiences. With regard to selecting which organisation to join, do not make a rushed decision. Instead, find out as much as you can about fees and services; most will offer reduced rates for students and joining incentives such as free nursing dictionaries. You may defer the decision until you have had time to discuss it with more senior students, staff in your placements or tutorial staff in the university.

SUMMARY OF KEY POINTS

- Starting to study as a student nurse can be challenging but the key to success is to be organised and well prepared.
- Get well prepared for study and be familiar with your timetable.
- Arrange your study area to make learning a comfortable and effective exercise.
- Take care of your health and safety as nursing can be physically demanding.
- Make time to read your handbooks so that you know where key policies are if you need them.
- Manage your written information by filing all important items carefully. You will need to refer to policies and guidelines at a later date.
- If you need help, ask for it as soon as possible. Remember that in the university there are a range of people from whom you can seek advice and guidance.

2

How to manage your time and study effectively

Learning outcomes

This chapter will help you learn how to:

- Motivate yourself to study
- Plan and use your time effectively
- Work out how much time you have to study
- Make the best use of your personal study time
- Explore ways to improve your ability to remember, concentrate and study more effectively
- Understand how you learn and your preferred learning style.

INTRODUCTION

When senior students were asked what advice they would give to those just starting, one commented, 'Plan to succeed'. Simply put, the statement says, if you want to succeed, then you almost certainly need to do some planning. When you are studying (we use the term studying to mean 'trying to learn', not just looking at printed material), you have many learning resources at your disposal (see Chapter 3). These resources range from people, such as tutors and librarians, to objects such as books and computers. However, the resource over which you have most control is your time.

Your time is yours to allocate as and how you like. There will, of course, be lots of things competing for your time; the trick is to decide how to allocate your time between these different things, how to make efficient use of that time and how to reduce your stress levels. There are two important points to remember: your time is yours to control and if you want to be a nurse, you must dedicate time to that goal.

When you start a pre-registration nursing course your life will change and, as a result, the way in which you use your time will also need to change. If you already have a busy life you will need to consider how you will adjust your life to accommodate your studies. The adjustments you make are likely to affect your friends and family, so it is a good idea to discuss this with them. One of the most important aspects of planning your time is to think about how you currently use time.

Time budgets

In order to accommodate a new learning experience you need to adjust how you currently spend your time so that you can allow time for the new activity. Think of the time that you have available as your time budget. In the same way as you can end up with no money if you do not budget your money carefully, you can end up with a crisis due to no time if you do not budget your time carefully. Think of the implications for your family and friends; changing your time budget may affect their time budget as well, so you may want to discuss your plans with them. If you do not think about planning your time now you may find later that you have a time crisis. There are 168 hours in a week. You will probably need to devote about 56 hours to sleeping, but how you manage the rest of your hours is up to you.

One way to start managing your time is to make a record of what you do with your time. Pick a typical week and keep a record of how you allocate your time over the week, perhaps using a method like the one shown in Table 2.1. Use abbreviations to indicate different activities; for example, T for travel, W for work, S for studying, E for eating, etc. You should consider including activities such as childcare, family commitments, leisure (TV, reading, etc.), personal care/hygiene, sleeping, sport/exercise and socialising.

To do this exercise effectively you need to complete the table at least once a day but it works best if you keep a diary as you go about your daily activities. When you change activities, record in your diary how much time you spent on the previous one. Now calculate how much time you spend in each activity. Are there any areas in your weekly schedule where you could make better use of your time? Once you identify how you currently spend your time you can start to plan how

Table 2.1 Time budget

Time	Mon	Tues	Wed	Thurs	Fri	Sat	Sun
00.00	Sl	Sl					
01.00	Sl	Sl					
02.00	Sl	Sl					
03.00	Sl	Sl					
04.00	Sl	Sl					
05.00	Sl	Sl					
06.00	S/E	S/E					
07.00	PC	PC					
08.00	T	T					
09.00	W	W					
10.00	W	W					
11.00	W	W					
12.00	W	W					
13.00	W	W					
14.00	W	W					
15.00	W	W					
16.00	W	W					
17.00	T	T					
18.00	CC/E	CC/E					
19.00	CC	CC					
20.00	L	L					
21.00	S	L					
22.00	S/E	S/E					
23.00	Sl	Sl					

Partially completed record of a time budget. Each box represents 1 hour of time; where there is more than one activity in a particular hour, more than one symbol has been entered.
CC, childcare; E, eating; L, leisure; PC, personal care; S, study; Sl, sleep; T, travel; W, work.

you will accommodate your studies. This technique can help you manage your time and stay in control of your life. For example, you may need to seek help with childcare, from family or friends, to enable you to study. Being in control of how you spend your time can help reduce the stress levels in your life.

There are some limitations to time management and these revolve around the fact that the way in which we perceive time and the tasks we have to do will depend on the circumstance. Take a look at two sayings connected with time and tasks:

'If you want something done ask a busy person'
(Anon)

'A job expands to fit the time available to it'
(Anon)

What these sayings suggest is that time is an unusual phenomenon, that some people seem to be able to achieve a lot more than others in the same amount of time, and that if we focus and concentrate on a task we can accomplish it in less time. This chapter is designed to help you focus and concentrate on your studies and help you to make the best use of whatever time you have for your studies.

MAKING GOOD USE OF YOUR STUDY TIME

When you start a full-time course (or even a part-time course) you will need to spend a considerable amount of time on your studies, so you will need to plan for this. Having put aside time for study in your schedule, you need to think about making the most of that time.

Managing your study time

As you get into your studies you are likely to find competing demands on your time. For example, you need to write up your lecture notes, complete assignments and reflect on practice. You need to think about how you will complete all you have to do so that you can succeed.

One method of time management is to prioritise tasks and design schedules or timetables. If you are a very spontaneous sort of person, learning schedules are probably not for you; however, you will still need to think about how to focus your attention on your priorities (see pp. 19, 22). When designing schedules you need to decide which tasks are the most important to achieve and when you will accomplish them.

Tasks are likely to include:

- attending lectures
- searching for information
- assignments
- presentations
- meetings with your tutor
- reading
- writing up notes
- reviewing notes, etc.
- studying
- seminar preparation
- planning/scheduling
- meetings with your mentor
- practising clinical skills
- reflection.

Schedules

One way to manage your study time is to use a series of schedules that relate to different periods of time and priority levels. Make a schedule of all the important

Table 2.2 Main tasks during the period January–April

Date	Main task
12 January	Collect essay guidelines
08 April	Assessment due
12 March	Martha's 60th birthday
19 March	Clinical exam
20 April	Go on holiday

tasks, indicate hand-in dates for all assignments and add other tasks as they occur (Table 2.2). Give yourself target dates for all tasks and indicate which are the most important. Remember the assignment hand-in date must not be your target date; you should aim to finish a week before the official hand-in date (see Chapter 6).

From the completion date of these tasks you should then work back to important points that lead to the completion of the task. If, for example, you need to produce an essay, an important point could be the completion of the search of the literature or delivering a first draft to your tutor (see Chapter 6). You need to add the suggested completion date to your schedule for each of these important points. When managing a project, these important points are often called milestones. Once all your milestones have been logged and given completion dates, you have your main schedule (Table 2.3).

Weekly schedule

The next level of planning is your weekly schedule, which should be informed by your main schedule but needs to include basic study tasks such as reviewing, practising, searching for information and a visit to your tutor. You may need to form weekly lists of tasks to inform your schedule, indicating which day you will complete each task (Table 2.4). Prioritise each task using EIC ('Essential', 'Important' and 'Can wait'). Essential tasks must be done that day. Important tasks have a high priority but not as high as Essential tasks. Can wait tasks can be put off. 'E' tasks need to have a firm time when they will be tackled: everything stops for an 'E'. 'I' tasks should also have a firm time, but 'C' tasks can be slotted in when time allows (but should not be put off forever). Cross tasks off your list as you complete them; this will give you a feeling of satisfaction and a sense of achievement.

When you form your schedule, allocate a certain amount of time to each task. In forming your weekly study schedule you need to bear in mind your overall time budget (see pp. 20, 21).

Tip

Use a notebook or diary for your planning schedule and always carry this with you. You can then use spare time while travelling to review your schedules and add/remove tasks. It is important not to spend so much time writing schedules that there is no time left to complete the task!

Table 2.3 Main schedule (January–April): Each milestone relates to a main task and signifies an activity that must be completed by the date specified in the left-hand column

| Due date | Main tasks and their milestones | | | |
	Essay	Martha's 60th	Holiday	Clinical exam
14th Jan	Note down initial thoughts			
04th Feb	Complete initial search for information			
10th Feb			Book holiday	Attend overview
12th Feb		Make invitation lists		
14th Feb		Send out invitations	Pay deposit	
25th Feb	Complete read through of information with notes	Buy present		Attend revision session
29th Feb	Finish essay plan – show tutor			Self test
8th March				Mock exam
10th March	Finish writing essay			Exam
12th March	Draft to tutor	Buy party stuff		
19th March	See tutor	PARTY		
08th April	Hand-in date			
20th April			Go on holiday	

Daily schedule

It is also a good idea to have a daily schedule. Look at your weekly schedule each night or morning to see what you were meant to have achieved and how well you have done. Then schedule your day, again using a list of the tasks you need to complete, and prioritising the tasks using the EIC system (see p. 19).

Review your schedules

You must make sure you review your schedules regularly or you may not meet an assignment deadline, or fail to revise sufficiently. Your review needs to be done both daily and weekly: on a daily basis look at what you didn't achieve or, if you feel you spent too little or too much time studying a particular subject, adjust the

Table 2.4 Weekly schedule* for 10–17 February showing the important events of the week with their priority using the EIC system

Monday	Make invitation list (E)	Write invitations (I)	Do shopping (I)	Attend overview (E)	Phone Mum (C)	Visit library (C)
Tuesday	Go to work (E)	Attend lectures (E)	Attend lectures (E)	Go to gym (C)		Visit library (C)
Wednesday	Send invitations (E)	Go out with friends (I)	Do washing (C)	Attend lectures (E)		Do some studying (C)
Thursday	Practise clinical skills (I)	Attend lectures (E)	Do ironing (C)	Go to gym (C)		Review study material (I)
Friday	Go to work (E)	Practise clinical skills (I)	Go out with friends (I)			Read two articles (I)
Saturday	Go to work (E)	Go out with friends (I)	Do shopping (C)			Review notes (I)
Sunday			Go to gym (C)	Friends round (I)	Cinema (C)	

Note that this schedule does not indicate how much time is allocated to each task and that the priority status of an activity will tend to increase the longer it is ignored.

next day's schedule. Your weekly review needs to do the same, but also needs to be based on an overall view of how long particular tasks take. The time you take to achieve tasks will change as you become more experienced and if tasks that you need to complete become more challenging. When you do a weekly review, you must also consider your overall schedule in order that you remain on target.

The 'Pickle Jar'

Another way of thinking about tasks and time is known as the Pickle Jar (Wright 2002) (Fig. 2.1). Here you imagine that all your available time is represented by a large empty jar and you first fill your jar with the big important tasks – the ones that are going to make a difference to your life and studies. Each task or aspect of your life or work is represented by a stone: big important tasks are the big stones and small tasks are the small stones. If you fill your jar with small 'stones' first, there is no room for the big 'stones'; however, if you fill your jar with big stones first you will notice that there is still space, and this space can be filled with the less important small stones. Thus, tasks such as answering the latest text message or email will probably come into the small stone category which should fit around your large stones, and not be dealt with first.

Using pictures

An alternative method is to draw a picture that shows your different goals and their importance to you. Within the picture the more important tasks will stand

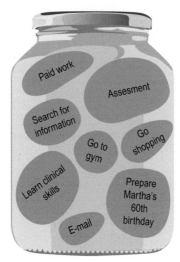

Figure 2.1 The Pickle Jar of time management

out and you can use this to help centre your thoughts and focus on which activities are most important.

Using spare time

Even with careful planning you may find that you have time in your day which is difficult to use; for example, time spent travelling or when waiting for a bus. It is a good idea to keep some study material to hand just for these times. Ideally, this should not be essential material but some of the additional reading required for most courses. Essential reading should be given serious study time. Similarly, try to always carry a notebook for recording questions and ideas as they come to mind. You can also use it to jot down any tasks that you suddenly remember you need to do, or thoughts and ideas you have for your next essay.

Use any small amounts of spare time between lectures to go over what you previously covered, note down what you understood from the previous lecture and what you feel you need to do more work on.

Improving your memory skills

Forgetting is a natural phenomenon and is probably designed to help keep our brains functioning correctly. While we might think that bright people don't forget, a study of members of the Psychological Society found that 2 weeks after a seminar more than 90% of the points raised in the seminar had either been forgotten or were remembered incorrectly (Hunter 1957, cited by Pauk 1993). Most people have perfectly good memories; if you have obtained the qualifications needed to get onto your nursing course, then your memory will be up to the job. Being absent minded is not the same as having a poor memory. Being unable to find your keys is not because you have a bad memory but because you did not pay attention to

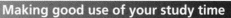

> ## Box 2.1 Some things that motivate
>
> - Desire to be a registered nurse
> - Desire to succeed
> - Need to prove one's self
> - Wanting to learn
> - Family pressure
> - Not wanting to fail
> - Desire to accomplish something
> - Desire to gain status
> - Fascination with a subject
> - Want to be an effective, safe, professional practitioner

where you put them in the first place. To remember something you must put effort into committing it to memory.

Psychologists do not really understand how or why we forget things but there are techniques that can help us to remember. Some techniques are linked to concentration and finding out how best we study; others attempt to help us structure information within our brains. The good news is that we can improve our memory. Psychologists conducting research into memory have suggested some of the following approaches.

Motivation

You will be amazed what you can learn and remember when you are motivated to do so. Research suggests that individuals can recall information much better when they are paid to remember or know they are going to be tested on what has been learned. When studying at university or college your motivation can come from a number of sources. Look at Box 2.1 and then think about the things that motivate you. Make your own list and pin it in a place where you will see it every day before you go to college or out to a practice placement. Doing this will help you to remember why you decided that you want to be a nurse and this will motivate you. The more you are motivated, the more you are likely to learn (see p. 31). Stress impairs your body's ability to remember, so cramming for exams the night before will not be effective, nor will trying to remember the ward's policy and procedures the day before you go on your placement.

> ### Tip
>
> If you are feeling stressed and worried about whether you have passed an exam or essay, this can distract you from getting on with other work and prevent you from enjoying and learning lots from your placement. Try writing down all your worries on a piece of paper, then fold up the paper and put it away in a drawer. Now try to actively put it out of your mind and focus on other things.

Understanding

Understanding is probably the best aid to memory; if you understand something you are much more likely to remember it. For example, if you are trying to remember how to measure blood pressure, you are much more likely to remember if you understand what you are trying to achieve and why each step is important.

Approaches to remembering facts and figures

There is no doubt that in order to succeed as a nurse you will need to be able to remember facts, figures and procedures. However, when it comes to procedures, you must understand what you need to do and why you are doing it, not simply trying to memorise it. In other words, remembering something is not the same as learning. Nevertheless, there will be times when you will want to focus on trying to remember. When you are trying to remember something, being able to concentrate is vital (see below).

Improving your memory skills depends on improving your overall mental functioning. To do this you need to exercise your brain; for example, try solving mental problems such as crosswords or Su Doku puzzles, or undertaking activities that stretch your mental abilities (e.g. playing chess). There are many books available which contain tests and challenges to exercise your brain (e.g. Mason & Kohn 2001). You also need to get plenty of sleep and eat a balanced diet. Research suggests that a diet rich in omega-3 fatty acids (found in fish oils) and low in saturated fat is good for brain functioning and overall health (Liebman 2002, Sinclair & Wesinger 2004). It is also wise to avoid excessive consumption of alcohol or the use of recreational drugs as these can seriously impair brain function.

Using mnemonics

As well as developing your brain function, there are also various techniques you can attempt when trying to remember specific items of information. Most of these techniques are based on the notion that our brains did not evolve to remember information that is written down or numbers, but evolved to work with information such as colours, three-dimensional structures and objects, spoken language, emotions, touch and smells. In other words, our memory is designed for the natural world of our ancestors. For example, one of the simplest ways to help remember text-based information is to read it out loud.

Most memory techniques designed for specific items of information involve linking the information that you want to remember to a form of information with which your brain prefers to work.

A common technique is to use a mnemonic. A mnemonic is a device, such as a verse, to improve memory. One of the most well know is the verse '30 days hath September, April, June and November' to remember the number of days in each month of the year. The idea here is that the memory is associated with the rhythm rather than just the information that is being remembered. Mnemonics do not need to be a rhyme. For strains and sprains, the recommended first aid is Rest, Ice, Compression and Elevation – this forms the acronym RICE. You may find this acronym alone helps you to remember the process. You can invent mnemonics

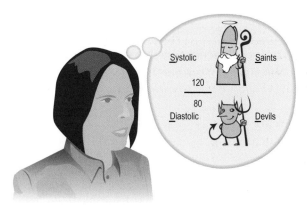

Figure 2.2 Saint (systolic) and devil (diastolic)

for any information you find difficult to commit to memory. If you use rhymes or acronyms, those that are funny, quirky or even rude seem to work better!

> ### Tip
> When remembering the risk assessment for moving and handling, use the mnemonic TILE, i.e. **T**ask, **I**ndividual (nurse), **L**oad (patient/item) and **E**nvironment.

Using images and feelings

Associations are another form of mnemonic. In an association you associate the thing you are trying to remember with an image or feeling. In general, the stronger the image, the more likely you are to remember. For example, when learning about blood pressure recording you need to remember that the systolic pressure is the top number and the diastolic pressure the lower number. To help remember which is which, you might think of Saints (S for systolic) are above Devils (D for diastolic) (Fig. 2.2).

The types of association that you make will depend on how your memory and imagination work. You can also use spatial memories to help. For example, if you have problems remembering the gross anatomy of the heart, you could imagine it as a two-up, two-down house set into a cliff where you enter at the top and leave from the bottom. The upper rooms represent the atria and the lower rooms the ventricles. The valves and vessels are doors.

There are numerous books that describe in more detail these and other memory techniques. If you want to learn more, we suggest reading O'Brien (2003).

Breaking up information

We tend to remember things better if the information is delivered in small amounts. Think for example of trying to remember telephone numbers; the longer the

Box 2.2 Try this – learning numbers

In turn, memorise each sequence so that you can recall it to a friend. Time how long it takes you to perfect each sequence.

a. 4 6 3
b. 7 9 5 3 2 9
c. 6 5 7 9 1 4 3 4 6
d. 8 7 4 6 3 2 3 1 7 9 8 2 3

telephone number, the harder it is to learn. Look at Box 2.2 and try to remember the different sequences of numbers. What happens as the sequence becomes longer?

You probably found that, as the number of digits increased, the time required to learn the numbers escalated. Thus, learning in small chunks is more efficient. This theory (Ebbinghaus 1885) also provides a good explanation as to why last minute revision and 'cramming' are so inefficient. When you are studying it is better to work with smaller chunks of information, breaking down a subject into sections. You may start with an overview of a subject, but then try to tackle smaller bits. For example, if learning the bones in the skeleton, first focus on a subsection such as the hand, the wrist, then the forearm and upper arm.

Grouping

Grouping similar aspects together can also help you to remember. For example, when shopping it is much easier to remember what you want to buy if you group similar items together under distinct headings such as fruit, vegetables, stationery, etc. With regard to nursing, if you are considering an activity such as hand hygiene you may group together aspects under headings such as 'my actions' and 'equipment I need'. If thinking of nursing assessments, you may want to group the things you need to assess under different aspects of well-being, such as physical, emotional and spiritual.

Visualisation

Trying to remember things as pictures or visual stories can help. For example, you could picture yourself actually doing the patient's blood pressure. To remember the pattern of blood circulation through the heart, you might imagine yourself as a blood corpuscle taking a journey through the circulation and noticing the structures as you go. Some people can also remember important facts by visualising them; for example, if you are trying to remember the concentration of normal saline, try to picture that concentration written clearly in big bold letters on the container (Fig. 2.3).

Using stories

Narrated stories are still used by many cultures as repositories of knowledge, information and understanding, particularly those cultures in which writing is relatively uncommon. Make up a story that depicts the thing you are meant to remember.

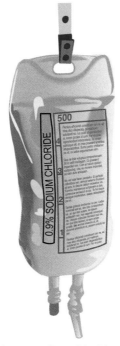

Figure 2.3 Bag of fluid labelled 0.9% sodium chloride

Box 2.3 **A story explaining some of the issues in relation to meticillin-resistant *Staphylococcus aureus***

The evil knight *Meticillin Resistant* rode on his horse *Staphylococcus aureus* causing much distress and injury among the *vulnerable* patients. Why has this *MRSA* (for that is what it is called) come to haunt us and why can't we see it and what can we do? This enemy, the elders explained, is 'very, very small, only visible under a microscope (*microscopic*) and is known as a *bacterium*'. It, they confessed, 'has become resistant to many of our weapons (*antibiotics*)'. This resistance had been caused by the overuse of antibiotics that resulted in the rapid *evolution* of *resistant strains* and high levels of cross-infection caused by patients living in *close proximity* and poor *hand hygiene* practice among the elders (who were seldom attacked by MRSA!).

Although the story does not need to make sense, it does need to be memorable. You can make up stories by taking the key words from the subject you are trying to remember and then link the words together in a story. Box 2.3 tells a story in relation to meticillin-resistant *Staphylococcus aureus*.

Concentrating while you study

Concentration is one of the keys to maximising what you learn in the time you devote to the process. It is important to identify how long you can study for before you stop being effective (20, 30 or 50 minutes?). You need to plan breaks in between your periods of study. Fill your breaks with non-study related activity such as making a cup of tea or doing domestic tasks like vacuuming or loading the washing machine, tasks that in themselves do not require much concentration. In these breaks, mull over what you have just learned or are going to write next.

If you are studying subjects that you find difficult, then you will probably be able to concentrate for a shorter period. Conversely, if your studying involves an activity such as searching for material or practising a practical skill, you will probably find that your ability to concentrate is extended. You need to identify how long you can maintain concentration during particular study activities as it will help you to allocate your time and identify how to use your breaks. Concentration can also be improved by using appropriate note-taking techniques (see Chapter 4). Consider your 'best' time to study. Most of us have a time when our biological clock is at its most effective and at these periods you will work best. For example, if you are a 'morning' person, getting up an hour earlier to study is likely to be much more productive than working late at night.

Healthy lifestyle

Concentration and memory can be affected by lifestyle. You need to make sure that you eat a balanced diet, take exercise and have enough sleep. Eating a balanced diet can sometimes be difficult if both your financial and time budgets are tight; it is a good idea to build time into your daily activities for meals and to try to maintain regular eating habits. There are a number of books that will show you how good food can be prepared on a tight budget. A good example is *More Grub on Less Grant: The New Student Cookbook* (Clarke 1999). This book has many ideas and costs very little.

Exercising is good for your health and your ability to cope mentally. Try to build exercise into your daily schedule. You could do this formally with activities such as going to a gym, swimming pool or playing sport, or informally such as walking or cycling to college. Exercising provides time for you and is a good way to reduce stress and anxiety.

> **Study Tip**
>
> Going for a brisk walk during a break in studying can provide useful thinking time as well as good exercise.

Having sufficient sleep is vital if you are to study effectively. You must plan to have about 7–8 hours of sleep per day. Less sleep than this will seriously affect your motivation and your ability to remember. Avoid substituting coffee (caffeine) for sleep; it does not work and if drunk in excess can cause anxiety. Unfortunately we cannot

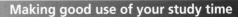
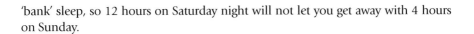
'bank' sleep, so 12 hours on Saturday night will not let you get away with 4 hours on Sunday.

> ### Tip
>
> To test whether you are getting enough sleep, darken your bedroom around mid-morning, set an alarm clock for 15 minutes and lie down. If the alarm clock wakes you up, you probably need more sleep; if you are perfectly awake when the alarm goes off, you are probably getting enough sleep or maybe more than you need (Pauk 1993).

Reducing distractions

Regardless of how you study, you need to be focused on what you are studying and to be free from things that distract you. What distracts us is very much an individual thing. Some people do not like studying in quiet rooms as they find silence distracting. Some writers suggest that you should set aside a place that you use specifically for studying (Pauk 1993) because if you only use that place for studying you are less likely to be distracted by other activities. Avoid bringing unnecessary objects such as photographs or ornaments into this place because they may distract you. Similarly, while natural light will help, if the view from the window is good you may find yourself spending too much time looking out of the window and not enough time at your books! Libraries tend to be good places to work as they are free from distractions. Some people like a TV or radio on in the background when they study, but this can be easily distracting, and it is important that you remember more about what you have studied than the TV programme.

Whatever your strategy, make sure that it works for you. You can do this by testing what you have learned from a period of study. Try to think about what you have learned immediately after a period of studying and also a few days later.

> ### Study Tip
>
> A personal stereo playing quiet instrumental or classical music can be useful in shutting out distracting noises such as people talking while you study.

Try out different environments for studying. Studying with friends and colleagues can be very effective and fun, but make sure it works. It is easy to think that you have spent several hours studying in the skills lab, practising how to measure blood pressure, when in fact 80% of that time was spent chatting with your friends.

Conditioning yourself

Conditioning yourself to study is another technique that is worth trying. Psychologists have learned that certain 'signals' can be used to stimulate certain behaviours.

The notion of conditioning was developed by a scientist called Pavlov who famously conditioned dogs to salivate when they heard a bell. Pavlov had trained the dogs to associate the sound of a bell with being fed; therefore when they heard the bell they salivated (Hill 1985). You can condition yourself to be in the mood to study. To do this you must consistently perform the same activity before you start studying; for example, listening to a certain piece of music. The conditioning will only be effective if you always start studying after that activity, so it is best not to choose a common activity such as making a cup of tea.

Distraction diary

One technique that will help you to develop your powers of concentration is to use a distraction diary. In a distraction diary, you keep a record of each time you lose your concentration and what distracted you. Sometimes this will be physical things such as being cold or hungry, sometimes alternative thoughts and sometimes worries or anxieties. Making a diary of these distractions will help you to identify specific factors that are distracting you. Having recognised these factors, you will be in a better position to do something about them. You must maintain your distraction diary while studying, not afterwards, because when you have lost concentration, using a distraction diary will help refocus your mind on your studies.

Not being able to concentrate can be an important signal about what you are studying in relation to your abilities. If you are studying something that is too difficult, anxiety and self-doubt will soon distract you. If, on the other hand, something is too easy you will soon become demotivated and bored. In both cases, you may want to seek the help of a tutor, friends or study group.

An alternative approach to distractions is to consistently ignore them; this can take real strength. When something first distracts, you may look up and take notice. The next time, you note it, but you insist to your mind that you will not respond. If you keep doing this, you will soon find that you can ignore the distraction; you can even train yourself to ignore the telephone.

Making lists

Concentration can also be improved by making a 'things to do' list and prioritising the tasks (see pp. 21, 22). Having this list will allow you to focus on what you are doing at the moment rather than being distracted by trying to remember the things you have not done. If you have allocated time to complete these things in your schedule (see p. 21), they will be even less distracting.

Getting started

Getting started on a new task or a new area of study can be difficult. We can find all sorts of reasons why not to start or other things to do. Too much of this type of delay can lead you into problems, so having some strategies to help in getting started is a good idea. Stop and think about the reasons why you are delaying getting started and write them down. Those that involve tasks can be allocated a new slot in your time schedule; other reasons such as 'because my friends aren't studying' will require you to challenge your overall motivation for wanting to study and to look at the sort of things that hold you back. Peer pressure not to study can be an issue and this is

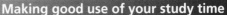

why forming and working in a study group can be really helpful. Once you are in a study group you will find that you will have peer pressure to study.

Make a plan to do specific items of study and stick to it. Be precise, for example: *I'm going to study the causes of heart disease tonight* rather than *I'm going to do some studying tonight.* A written note is harder to resist than a thought, so it is also a good idea to note in your diary or on a checklist what you plan to do. Using a schedule of intended study is a particularly good idea when you are revising for exams (see p. 21).

The 5-minute plan

If you are still having difficulties getting started, you could try the 5-minute plan suggested by Knaus (1997). Here you need to decide that you will do some studying or work on an assignment for just 5 minutes. Say to yourself, *I'll just do it for 5 minutes.* Five minutes is a small amount of time and does not seem like a great commitment. Before long you will find you have started the task and will probably carry on much longer than 5 minutes. Once the activity has been started, it will be much easier to get into the next time and eventually to finish.

Reviewing what you have learned

When studying it is important to build in review periods, where you put your study materials aside and really think about what you have learned during your last period of study. You can review what you have learned during a break, while you exercise or even on the bus. You should also be prepared to test yourself. This is important for information that you need to remember or for making sure that you can perform a procedure correctly. Most importantly, if your study strategy is working, you feel an increase in your confidence and probably an increase in your interest in your subject, which in turn will make studying easier.

Motivation

When you are studying on a course that extends over a number of years it is natural for your enthusiasm to go up and down. In the moments when your enthusiasm is low you may need to remotivate yourself. This is where motivation techniques can be of use. Lack of motivation often manifests itself in 'putting-off' behaviours. For example, the assignment and searching the research material can be 'put-off' to another day. This is known as procrastination. When we procrastinate we avoid engaging with a particular task, often by doing another. Sometimes students will avoid actually writing an assignment or essay by searching for material, constantly putting off the seemingly more unpleasant task.

One of the most important elements of becoming motivated is to spot when you are procrastinating. One way to do this is through examining what happens when you plan to do a task on a certain date: ask yourself whether you achieved the task on that date. Examine your planning schedule (see p. 21). What did you put off? Why did you put it off? If you put the activity off once it may be because you genuinely had to do something more important or did not feel up to the task, but if you kept putting it off you need to think about motivation.

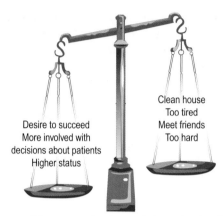

Figure 2.4 Weighing up different motivating and demotivating forces

Sometimes lack of motivation may be linked to not wanting to do a particular activity (e.g. essays); other times it is more general and because we lose sight of our purpose or goals. The latter tends to be more serious than the former.

Balancing

When thinking about a particular task there are forces that motivate us to do the task and also those that motivate us not to do it (Fig. 2.4). Some of these forces are internal (e.g. when we complete the task we will feel good about ourselves), while sometimes the motivation is external (e.g. when we complete the task we will be praised). Motivational forces can be positive or negative; for example, being fired if we do something wrong is a negative motivational force that drives us to do things right. Praise, on the other hand, is a positive force that also drives us to do things right.

The specific things that motivate us vary from individual to individual. When the forces to motivate us to do a particular task are outweighed by forces to do something else, we will tend to do the other thing. We quite often leave things we don't like doing to just before the deadline because it is only at this point that the motivational force to complete the task becomes very strong (e.g. failing an assignment if you don't hand it in). If you do find yourself procrastinating, it is a good idea to write down what motivates you. Start by answering questions such as:

- Why are you doing your course?
- What assignments do you prefer doing?
- Why do you prefer these?
- What do you want to achieve?

Rewards

When it comes to specific tasks such as assignments, many people find that rewards often help. Rewards can be particularly strong motivators if, in conjunction with a reward, you use a written contract. You must write the contract saying exactly what you are going to do and when (goals) and also clearly indicate what your reward will be (e.g. night out with friends). Tell people about your plan and make sure the reward is tangible. With things like assignments it is also important to view them as leading towards your long-term goals.

If you find studying hard because you lose sight of your goals, you may want to use things that constantly remind you of what you are trying to achieve. For example, if you want to make your goal visual, take a photograph of you in a nurse's uniform and pin it to your wall. The more real the image looks, the more it will help. Issues of motivation can also be linked to tiredness. If you are tired your motivation will fall, and the only solution will be to establish good sleeping habits. High levels of self-esteem are also linked to high levels of motivation.

> ## Tip
>
> When your motivation is flagging, picture yourself walking across the stage at graduation with all your friends and family cheering and applauding. Or imagine yourself as a registered nurse and answering the telephone saying, 'staff nurse speaking'. Keep these pictures in your mind.

Self-esteem

Self-esteem is your own assessment of your worth or value. Many of us are quite self-critical; this lowers our self-esteem and can lead to lower motivation. This is particularly so if a belief in our ability to self-develop is not strong. Self-esteem can be improved by challenging our own self-critique. The first stage in doing this is to articulate out loud or write down the self-critique that often occurs in our heads (sometimes called self-talk). Then, for each negative item, think of a positive item to counter or challenge it. Avoid dwelling on negative items. Remember you are in control of your own self-esteem – it is yours and you are making the judgements.

Think of all the positive things you have achieved in your life and let these form your opinion of yourself. Take time to congratulate yourself on what you have achieved. As your self-esteem rises, you will develop an increased sense of control of your life and with it an increase in motivation. Your increased motivation will lead to you achieving more and thus an increase in self-esteem, thereby creating a virtuous circle. If you believe that you have low self-esteem and that it is affecting your studies, you should seek advice from your university's counselling services. Two useful sources of information on self-motivation are the website www.unisanet. unisa.edu.au/motivation, and *100 Ways to Motivate Yourself* (Chandler 2004).

THINKING ABOUT HOW YOU LEARN (LEARNING STYLES)

Research suggests that we all prefer to learn in different ways (Dunn et al 1995) but often do not stop and think about how we like to learn. Establishing how you like to learn may help you to learn more efficiently and may explain why you enjoy some learning activities more than others.

People vary in the way that they like to perceive new information, how they like to process that information and the way that they approach any particular item of learning (Felder 1993). At university it is unlikely that your tutors will always cater for your learning style, but knowing your style might help you during periods of personal study and may help when in practice placements. Thinking about how you like to learn will probably help you to learn, simply because you have started to think about the process of learning. The process of learning involves perceiving information and then processing that information.

Perceiving information

We perceive information through our senses (sight, hearing, smell, taste and touch). When we learn, we use all of our senses but we will have a preference for receiving information visually (pictures, diagrams), aurally (sounds, words) or kinaesthetically (movement, touch) (Gardner 1993).

Visual learners

If you are a visual learner you will pick up information from pictures and diagrams easily; you will also tend to learn quickly from demonstrations and displays (Dunn & Dunn 1978). It would seem logical that people with a preference for visual learning would also like to learn from text. However, educational psychologists have noticed that when we read we tend to convert the text to words we listen to in our minds. Thus, while reading may appear to be a visual function, those who prefer aural learning tend to be those who most like learning from text.

Aural learners

Aural learners enjoy talk-based lectures and any situation where the information is spoken. Aural learners tend to enjoy discussion and debate and they will also tend to remember spoken information well. Some auditory learners like to talk to themselves or others as they learn. Other aural learners will continue the dialogue in their minds and think back on the words of others (Dunn & Dunn 1978).

Kinaesthetic learners

Kinaesthetic learners tend to prefer learning by doing, but also tend to want to move around as they learn. Kinaesthetic learners are much more likely to remember after having done something rather than having read about it. Kinaesthetic learners enjoy acting out scenarios, labs and practical classes. If you are a kinaesthetic learner you will find it difficult to remember how to do a particular procedure until you have done it (Dunn & Dunn 1978).

Once you have identified your dominant learning style you may want to tailor some of your learning activities to suit it (Table 2.5). Do be aware, however, that you will inevitably be required to engage with a variety of different learning materials throughout your career. Over-focussing on your preferred style may not help you if it is not that which dominates your field of study and, no matter how much you love or hate it, reading is something that all students have to do.

Table 2.5 Learning activities that suit particular learning styles

Kinaesthetic	Aural	Visual
Move around as you study	Talk about the thing you are learning	Draw the issue
If trying to understand the rationale for a process, try actually doing the process or using a model	Tape lectures to listen to them again	Use mind maps
Use models (computers or 3D) and simulations	Recall facts out loud	Watch a video
Go over what you are studying while doing other activities, e.g. swimming, washing-up	Focus you mind on what was being said during a lecture	Highlight important points in books in colour
Note taking	Reading	Use models

Adapted from Felder (1993) and Smith (2001).

Processing information

There are a number of differing styles when it comes to processing information; there are also a number of different schemes for classifying these styles. One of the most well known is that devised by Honey and Mumford (1992), who classified people into theorists, pragmatists, relativists or activists.

- *Theorists* like to know why things occur and happen; they try to put experiences into new theories and to relate their experience to existing theory.
- *Activists* tend to like doing things in order to learn; doing could be as simple as making notes or actively reading. They like new problems and challenges but have a preference for application and doing rather than observing.
- *Reflectors* like to take time to consider things, and are reluctant to give an answer straight away. They like to observe and research before reaching conclusions; reflectors tend to draw their own conclusions and are concerned to find out the truth.
- *Pragmatists* like to know and understand what works, and often do not appreciate abstract theory. They tend to like to know experts they can emulate. Pragmatists like to work with real problems and to try things out.

Honey and Mumford's classifications are similar to those of Kolb (1984). However, Kolb suggested that these styles occur as part of a learning cycle (Fig. 2.5) and that, although we all have a natural tendency to like a particular style, we all need to be able to move through the cycle.

Kolb's ideas relate well to nursing because his research concerned learning from experience. The implication from Kolb's work is that we need to work with styles that we are uncomfortable with in order to learn from our experience. Kolb termed the stages in the learning cycle and the corresponding approaches to learning as follows: concrete experience (pragmatist), reflective observation (reflector), abstract

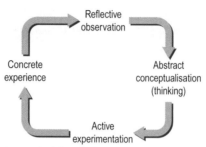

Figure 2.5 Kolb's learning cycle (after Kolb 1984, adapted from Jenkins 1998)

conceptualisation (theorist) and active experimentation (activist). In nurse education programmes you will be expected to perform all the stages of Kolb's cycle.

Learning from other approaches/styles

Adjusting the way you prefer to learn is probably not really possible, but learning more from other approaches probably is. To do this you need to be prepared to experiment and to engage. For example, if you are a theorist and do not like doing role play, the best way to get something from such an activity is to really focus on the fact that you are learning and to think about what you want to get out of the activity before you start. If you are not a natural reflector, using a structured framework for reflection may help (see Chapter 8). During lectures and tutorials, try to 'translate' the material into the form that you understand best. To develop a different learning style, try looking at the material using an approach with which you are less comfortable. Practise approaching lectures in another way and be open to a new way of learning. Try to adapt to your lecturer's style and see if this makes a difference to what you learn.

SUMMARY OF KEY POINTS

- Using a time schedule can help you make the best use of your study time.
- Using memory techniques such as mnemonics can help you recall key facts and figures; however, understanding a topic is the best aid to memory.
- Maintaining a healthy lifestyle, exercising and getting enough sleep will make it easier to concentrate when studying.
- Getting started can be the hardest part. Making 'to do' lists and 'just doing 5 minutes' can help you get started.
- Picturing yourself as a registered nurse or on graduation day can help when your motivation to study is flagging.
- Understanding your preferred learning style will help you during periods of personal study and when on clinical placements.

3

Learning resources

Learning outcomes

This chapter will help you understand:

- What learning resources are available
- How to use handbooks and reading lists
- Which books to buy
- Where to find information
- How to work with your personal tutor
- How study groups can help you learn
- Who can help you learn in your clinical placements.

USING LEARNING RESOURCES

When faced with the challenge of finding information for essays and exams you need to be able to make the best use of learning resources to help you learn effectively and efficiently. Learning resources are specific devices, services or people who can assist you to learn. As an independent or self-directed learner you will need to make best use of the resources available to help you with your studies. This chapter will focus on libraries, books, journals, computer-based materials, librarians, lecturers, the internet, placement staff, patients and other students.

To gain a breadth of knowledge you should use a wide range of resources to aid your studies. The university will provide resources such as the library, clinical skills laboratories and biology laboratories, and there are usually learning resources available in placement areas. You will also need to establish your own collection of materials from journals, the internet and the media as well as books. Your local library, as well as those provided by professional bodies such as the Royal College of Nursing (www.rcn.org.uk), can be another source of information.

How to get started

Keep a special notebook for all information sources. Make notes in sessions designed to introduce you to the university library and study skills sessions. Important things to record are access times, borrowing regulations, recommended books and internet sites. Remember to save the addresses of good internet sites, just as you should always make a note of and file the details of good books.

Course handbooks

You will be given a lot of written information when you commence your programme. Skim read these to find out what they contain (see p. 84 for reading techniques). Some of this information will provide advice or guidance on how to learn effectively, so file them carefully for future reference as you are very likely to need this information again.

Key information about your programme or module will normally be provided in the form of a handbook. Keep yours with all your other learning resources, as you may need to refer to them when completing your assignments. These will detail all university policies. Separate handbooks may be provided for modules and programmes and these will detail course content, assessment guidelines and reading lists. Many universities provide handbooks online for you to download.

Reading lists

Reading lists are often provided in student handbooks at the start of a programme. These can contain long lists of books and may look daunting but you are certainly not expected to read all the books listed. Reading lists are intended to help you start selecting appropriate books and are likely to contain materials available in the university library. Remember that textbooks are not intended to be read from cover to cover like a novel. Find out from the lecturers which books are considered as essential as this will help you prioritise your choice of reading. Don't confine yourself to books only on the reading list. There may be other good alternatives written in a style that you prefer.

University staff

The university staff employed to help you include course administrators, specialist teachers, computer support staff, programme leaders and your personal tutor.

Course administrators

The organisation of your course is likely to be dealt with by course administrators. Their role will include handling applications, completing joining papers, helping to organise your uniform and placements, and managing the assessment process. You will probably need to contact the course administrators when you have specific issues, such as if you change your address. If you have bursary issues the administrators will be able to give you contact details of the relevant people. They can also put you in touch with those who can help with financial issues and benefits advice (see pp. 12, 127). Most universities will have a 'help desk' system as the first point of contact for most queries.

Programme tutors

There will be a designated team of tutors who will work together to manage the academic side of your programme of study. It is a good idea to make note of their names and roles so that you know who to contact if you have any urgent issues. The different sections of your course (e.g. modules or units of the programme) may be the responsibility of certain tutors who will be able to help with specific aspects and issues in relation to their part of your course.

Specialist teachers

Subject specialists are the teaching staff you will meet in your lectures and seminars and you may feel that you need their advice or help in developing your understanding of their subject area. These lecturers will be able to direct you to specific learning materials. Academics have many demands on their time so it is best to make an appointment rather than just turning up at their office door. Do not be afraid to ask but do make sure you are prepared with specific questions and be clear about which aspects of the lecture you did not understand.

Keep records of your lecturers' names and the subjects that they teach in case you need to contact them. You may be able to check the university website for teachers if you need to contact them at a later date.

Learning support tutors

Most universities provide additional academic support for students who need extra help in acquiring academic skills and those with dyslexia or other special needs. You may be referred to such a service by your personal tutor or you may be able to self refer if you think you need extra help. These units may also have advisors trained to deal with dyslexia; if you think you may have a problem with reading and writing, seek advice. Use these facilities to help you develop your study skills and maximise your learning; that is what they are there for. Don't feel embarrassed to ask for help.

There may also be special classes for students for whom English is a second language or for students who have not had recent experience of writing essays or sitting exams. It is important that you use these group sessions, as working with other students may be helpful for some aspects of academic writing.

IT support teachers

As a nurse you will need information technology (IT) skills for record keeping, data analysis and nursing records. If you are not familiar with using computers you must take every opportunity to learn. Most universities have IT support teachers who will provide training and will also provide you with user guides and manuals. Your university may offer the IT qualification the European Computer Driving Licence (www.ecdl.com) to enable you to reach the required level of proficiency in IT skills. Completing assignments will help you develop IT skills and will also save you time. You will find that many of your tutors taught themselves and struggled initially. In fact, some of us were there at the beginning when computers were first introduced!

Tip

If you are not familiar with word processing, do this for your first essay. You are likely to have more spare time at the beginning of the course and if your computer skills are limited this is when you should learn. It will save you time later.

Your personal tutor

Your university will allocate you a personal tutor who is appointed to provide you with academic support and guidance. Your personal tutor will be able to advise you on your personal plan of study. In some universities the personal tutor will also provide pastoral support (advising you on personal issues which may be affecting your studies); in others the pastoral and academic roles will be separate.

It is important to remember that your tutors are human, and as such their personalities and ways of working will vary. As well as being lecturers, they are usually registered nurses (or other health care professionals) and many will have clinical commitments as well as their university role. Your relationship should be productive, but if you are unhappy with your personal tutor, check your course/university handbook for advice. Your personal tutor is there to help but will not organise your study time for you. Tutors want their students to succeed; it gives them a nice 'glow' inside.

Taking responsibility for your own learning

As an adult you will be expected to be responsible for your own learning; however, this does not mean you have to do it all by yourself and that no one will help you.

Box 3.1 Checklist for your first meeting with your personal tutor

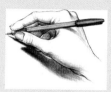

- Name and title of your personal tutor – find out how they like to be addressed
- Their office location
- Exchange contact details – telephone number, fax number and email address
- Find out good times to call and when they are planning to be away
- Agree the general frequency of meetings
- Agree times and methods for submitting draft essays
- If your tutor is difficult to contact, make the next appointment each time you meet

---

Being responsible for your own learning means making the best use of learning opportunities, organising your own study time and ensuring that you plan your work and assess your own progress.

Frequency of meetings with your personal tutor

Your tutor will advise you how often you need to meet; universities will normally suggest a minimum number of meetings per term or semester (Box 3.1). Make use of alternative forms of contact such as telephone tutorials and email; when you contact your personal tutor, always be ready to leave a voicemail message in case they are not able to take your call.

Study Tip

If leaving a voicemail message for your personal tutor, speak clearly, stating your name, the reason for your call and your telephone number – it is a good idea to repeat the number. Always leave your number even if you know that your tutor has a record of it. Your tutor may not be in their office when they listen to your message.

If using your university email system, your computer log-in 'name' is often a number so remember to include your full name in the email.

Tutorial records for your portfolio

Good record keeping skills are essential in nursing and you should start this as a student. Keep a record of your contact with your personal tutor for your portfolio as this will show that you are able to use appropriate support systems in your professional career. It may also be useful if you have to write an essay about your personal development throughout the course; notes of your personal tutor meetings can jog your memory.

Phone or online tutorials

As an alternative to a face-to-face meeting, your personal tutor may be happy to discuss issues on the telephone. Remember to take notes and keep a record of the date. Some tutors may be able to chat 'online' or use electronic message boards, but this sort of communication does not suit all academics.

Group tutorials

A number of your colleagues may have the same personal tutor or if a group of you have the same sort of questions it is often beneficial to meet with your tutor as a group. This saves the tutor having to repeat things and you may find it easier to share your concerns. Tutors do appreciate this sort of initiative and group tutorials can prove to be helpful as your colleagues may ask questions that you had not considered.

Draft essays

Assignments are learning experiences and you should use your personal tutor to comment on your work in progress (Box 3.2). You need to submit a draft to your

---

Box 3.2 Your personal tutor

Things your personal tutor will expect from you:

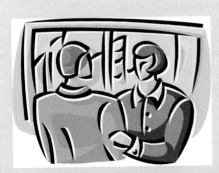

- To be motivated to learn and try hard to succeed
- To complete any learning activities that they might give you
- To maintain regular contact
- To inform them of any important issues or changes, e.g. if you move house or suffer a family bereavement
- To be prepared for planned meetings
- To attend meetings and to arrive at the designated time

Things you can expect from your personal tutor:

- To be knowledgeable and enthusiastic about nursing
- To be respectful and to discuss (although not always agree with) alternative views
- To be able to understand the student's perspective – they were students once
- To give you their time
- To read through and give timely feedback on your draft assignments
- To direct you to extra academic support if it is required
- To be able to either provide or know where to find help if you have a personal issue
- To give praise and encouragement

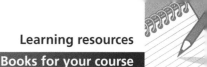

tutor at least 4 weeks before the submission date to give them time to make comments and return it to you while there is still time for you to act on their advice. If you are meeting with your personal tutor to discuss a draft essay, send them the draft a few days before the meeting. That way your tutor will have time to read the essay before you meet, rather than during your meeting.

Remember, your personal tutor is there to help you but cannot do it for you. They are not there to say whether your essay is good enough to pass, and most will not read final essays for this reason. Your tutor is there to help you develop your ideas and your academic style, and to make sure that you are following the assessment guidelines.

Study Tip

In order to maintain a good working relationship with your personal tutor:

- **Do** keep appointments and arrive on time. Ensure you telephone if it is not possible for you to attend. If you arrive late, they will not be able to spend as much time with you.
- **Do** leave clear voicemail messages – always state your full name, course details and telephone callback details (repeating the telephone number is helpful).
- **Do** ask for help when you need it. Do not wait until it is too late.
- **Do** be prepared for tutorials – take all relevant documents with you and write down questions you wish to ask.
- **Do** make appointments to see your personal tutor on a regular basis.

BOOKS FOR YOUR COURSE

The books that you will need range from large tomes to small pocket guides. The larger books are sometimes referred to as textbooks as they are for specialist study rather than general non-fiction. Many of these large textbooks are edited books. The chapters in an edited book are often written by different authors and their names will be at the beginning of the chapter or in the contents list. The arrangement of these chapters is then done by the editor(s) and it is their name(s) that appear on the cover. Occasionally an edited book will not have named chapter authors, usually because a large number of people have contributed to the book.

You may be familiar with English language dictionaries which explain words but you will also need to use subject dictionaries such as nursing or psychology. These are useful for finding definitions of a subject to help you start an essay, understand a term that you have found in another book or something you have heard while on placement. A pocket size nurses' dictionary is essential when starting in placement.

Buying books

Textbooks are an essential resource for any course and good ones will become valued and treasured. Family and friends may offer to buy you books when you start your course but it's best to check out a range of books before you spend your money, unless you are instructed to purchase a set book. Wait until you have discussed your needs and have had a chance to look at the texts available before making your choices. In order to use your money wisely it is best to discuss your options with tutors, librarians and other students before you buy books. Students who are ahead of you on the programme and those who have just completed it can be very informative; they will tell you which books they found most useful. They may offer to sell you their books but be careful; nursing and health care change rapidly and clinical books quickly become outdated.

When buying a book there are a number of questions you need to ask:

- *How up to date is the book?* This is indicated by the publication date of the book. In some subjects, having an up-to-date edition is very important, e.g. clinical issues, drugs and pharmacology. Don't spend your money on out-of-date books.
- *How popular is the book?* The popularity of a book is a measure of how useful the book may be to you. Books that have been reprinted frequently and those with a number of editions are normally very popular. In the library, popular books are more likely to be out on loan or always on the 'returns' trolley rather than on the shelves. It is a good idea to check the 'returns' trolley regularly.
- *When was the most recent edition published?* Some of the popular textbooks are revised every 3–4 years. It's annoying to spend a lot of money buying a book only to find shortly afterwards that there is a new edition. If a popular book has not been revised in the last 5 years, a new edition is likely to be published soon. Check on the publisher's website to see if a new edition is about to be published. Your tutor may also be able to advise you whether to wait for a new edition.
- *Where was it written?* It is important when you buy a book that you are aware of the country or market for which it was written. This is significant in relation to the style of English and to legal and professional issues. Be careful, because terminology and practice differ from country to country. The place of publication is the important thing, not where it was printed. The place of publication is usually indicated on the title page or inside the front cover (Fig. 3.1).
- *How much does it cost?* An expensive book may be worth every penny if you use it a lot. Some textbooks are very expensive so seek advice from your tutors; it may be better to borrow them from the library first. Popular books may be a worthwhile buy as they are often not available in the library as someone else always gets there first. Having a comprehensive textbook (one that is recommended in your handbook is best) means that you can make a start on most essays at home. Carrying large books to and from the library may not be good for your back, so having your own copy is a good idea.

Essential Nursing Skills

SECOND EDITION

Maggie Nicol
BSc(Hons) MSc PGDipEd RGN
Senior Lecturer, Clinical Skills

Carol Bavin
DipN(Lond) RCNT RGN RM
Lecturer

Shelagh Bedford-Turner
RGN BSc(Hons) MSc(Nursing) DipN(Cert Ed)
Lecturer

Patricia Cronin
BSc(Hons) MSc(Nursing) DipN(Lond) RGN
Senior Lecturer

Karen Rawlings-Anderson
BA(Hons) MSc(Nursing) DipN Ed RGN
Senior Lecturer

 Mosby

EDINBURGH LONDON NEW YORK OXFORD PHILADELPHIA ST LOUIS SYDNEY TORONTO 2003

Figure 3.1 Book title page showing place of publication

- *Is the content clear?* Check the book's contents page to get a general idea of the range of topics covered and then try looking up some specific items in the index that you know are part of your course and may come up in assignments. If you can find these easily and the information is clear and concise, then the book is likely to be useful. A book with a glossary of terms may be particularly helpful.

Useful books to purchase

As discussed earlier (see pp. 43, 44), you should not rush into buying lots of books but the following are likely to be useful at the beginning of your course.

- A nursing dictionary – this will be particularly useful for placements. Some unions or professional bodies give these away if you join their organisation. If you need to consult a larger dictionary, use one in a library.
- If a subject is new to you (e.g. sociology) you may find a specific dictionary for that subject useful. There should be reference copies in the library to give you some idea of what is available.
- A comprehensive nursing skills book related to your branch or specialist area of study. Make sure it is up to date with current research. Look at the references at the end of the book or chapters and see if they mostly include recent publications within the previous 10 years. A number of suitable books should be recommended in your course handbook (see p. 38).
- A general nursing textbook, written for student nurses, which covers issues such as professional behaviour, legal issues, ethics, and health and safety, and explores the branches of nursing. This type of book may state that it is particularly suitable for the foundation programme. Ensure you are using a recent edition, one that refers to the Nursing and Midwifery Council (NMC), rather than the United Kingdom Central Council (UKCC), as the current controlling body for nurses and midwives.
- A biology book that you find easy to understand and again, a recent text is essential. Your biology lecturers can give advice on a book that is appropriate for your level, especially if you are new to the subject.
- Study skills books relevant to your needs. You may need a book that can help with grammar or, if English is not your first language, a book aimed at overseas students may be useful.
- Specialist study books can be an aid to studying a new subject (e.g. science) and help you understand the basic principles.

Study Tip

Ask you tutors: 'If you were only allowed to recommend one book, what would it be?' This may give you an idea of which book might be the first to consider buying.

Editions and reprints

Information about the edition or published version of a book is usually stated on the front cover unless it is a first edition (see Fig. 3.1). A second or subsequent edition is when the text is edited and revised. Over time the author's ideas may have changed or new legislation introduced so there is often a need to update books. It will usually state the date of the edition of a book on the bibliography page with all the details of printing, publishing and copyright, as well as dates of previous editions, if any.

Reprints are different from editions. A reprint means that the text has not been revised but that another batch of the same book has been printed. This may indicate that the book has become popular. You do not need to include information about reprints when referencing an essay (see Chapter 6), just the date of publication.

Buying second-hand books

Second-hand books might be useful but you should apply the same questions as you would to purchasing a new book. Libraries often have sales when they are replacing old stock. A newer edition will often say what material has changed in the book and it is always important to check this out. Remember that you may lose marks in your essay if you use out-of-date material.

> ### Tip
>
> For referencing purposes, only the second edition onwards is noted; therefore do not write 1st edition in your reference list. If you are unsure about publication details, ask the librarian for help.

Reading textbooks

Reading a textbook is not like reading a novel which you might read from cover to cover. You are much more likely to read only a relevant section or chapter of a book. When you decide to take out a book from the library, select one chapter or part of a chapter to read and take notes from it as soon as possible, preferably on the day you borrow it. Then you will have probably made the best use of the book. It's quite likely that you will not look at the book again until it is time to return it to the library. When selecting information to learn from a book, use the contents and index to search for specific items or chapters. Do not become despondent if you do not understand it straight away. You may need to read some parts more than once and then shut the book and try to explain to yourself what you have just read to check that you understand. If it's still unclear, you could discuss it with your colleagues at a study group or with your tutor. Trying to read it again the next day may also help, or you could try another textbook that explains it in a different way. Reading sections out loud can help you to remember.

> ### Study Tip
>
> When you borrow a library book, decide exactly which chapter or pages you will read first. Be realistic with regard to how much of a book you will read or you may be put off reading it at all. This way you will be making good use of the books you borrow from the library and not find yourself returning books you have never even opened.

Journals

Journals are formal, written publications that look like magazines. There are a huge number of nursing journals, from general nursing to highly specialist subject areas, and increasingly these are available via the internet. Your university library will have a subscription and you should be given a password to enable you to access them in the library. Check with your library to see whether you are able to access these journals via the internet from home.

The advantage of journals over books is that the articles, which are often recent research, are peer reviewed. This means that prior to publication a number of other experts in that particular field evaluate the article. Therefore the material in the article has been to some extent validated; this is important as not all research is of the same quality.

You should try to read at least one of the popular nursing journals on a regular basis to keep up to date with current debates and professional issues. The library will have copies but you may choose to buy a personal copy. You may like to keep some of the articles to use when writing assignments and will need to file these so you can find them later. One way to spread the cost of journals is to share them among your classmates.

Journals provide up-to-date information and the most recent research in nursing. In order to search for such information, you will need to use one of the computerised databases (see p. 62).

Computers and software

Although an in-depth knowledge of computers is not essential, you must be competent with regard to managing computerised information and should be able to produce your assignments using a word processor. Nurses must be IT literate and you must take all opportunities to learn how to use these as an aid to your learning. If you wish to purchase computer software to help you manage information (e.g. packages which arrange and store your references), or indeed a computer, there is likely to be a computer shop in the university that will sell these items at a competitive price and provide free advice.

Libraries and librarians

Libraries contain a variety of resources, such as books, journals, CD-ROMs, computer databases, search tools and librarians. Don't confine yourself to the nursing libraries; the main university library usually has a wider range of books on subjects such as sociology, psychology and biology. Your local public library can be a useful source of books as well as a quiet place to study. Other libraries, such as those of professional bodies like the Royal College of Nursing, can provide an alternative source of information and the health care trusts that provide your practice placements may also have libraries that you can use. This can be especially useful when you finish a shift and can fit in an hour's studying before going home.

Early in your course you should explore the printed resources available in the various libraries by spending time just looking through sections, becoming familiar with the range of textbooks and journals. Next, try to find some items that are linked to your current area of study and placement, and make some brief notes about the items you have found. This exercise can help you become familiar with your libraries and will save time in the future.

Librarians are experts at finding information. Check out whether they provide leaflets and other information designed to help you make the best use of the library resources.

Library fines and how to avoid them

If you fail to return items borrowed from the library you will accumulate fines. Ways to prevent this are:

- When you borrow an item, put a reminder of the date it is due back in your diary or on your mobile phone.
- Overnight, 3- and 7-day loans – check to see whether there are other copies available with longer loan periods.
- Don't borrow more books than you can realistically handle.
- Make sure you know the procedure for book renewals – this can often be done on the telephone or via the internet. However, do not count on being able to renew books; you may not be able to do this if someone else has requested it.

If you accumulate too many fines you may be barred from further borrowing until they are paid off. It may end up being cheaper to buy the books if your fines are extensive.

Librarians

Librarians are information location experts who are there to help you get the best from the library. They are usually busy so it's a good idea to think through what you want before you approach them with a question. Librarians can show you how to access the library catalogue and databases to search for information, and can help you refine your search and find what you are looking for (see Chapter 4, p. 62 for guidance on searching). Knowing what you want is a skill that will develop by listening carefully in lectures, reading your notes afterwards and checking your understanding by questioning yourself. For example, if you want to find information concerning communication skills, the librarians will find it easier to help you if you make it more specific, e.g. 'non-verbal communication' or 'communicating with patients who have communication difficulties'.

Studying in a library

Working in the library can be more productive than studying at home because there are fewer distractions. The time spent studying in a library tends to be better planned and therefore more efficient. Learning resources are at your fingertips and you can compare a number of texts. When planning your study for the week, you should aim to spend some of the time in the library. That way you may not need to borrow so many books as you can read and take notes in the library (Box 3.3). You can also plan some browsing time in the library to look through journals.

Box 3.3 Making notes in the library

When studying in the library, always make a note of the full details of the reference in case you require it for your essay. It could save you hours later:

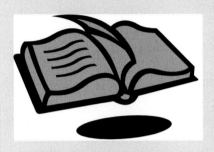

- Note the author(s) last name and initials
- Chapter author(s) and editor(s) if it is an edited book (see p. 43)
- Date of publication
- Title of book and edition or title of journal
- Journal volume and issue number
- Place of publication and publisher for books
- Page numbers – if it is a direct quote or if you wish to consult the book another time. To help you locate the book or journal again it is a good idea to make a note of which library it was in and the shelf reference number, which is usually on the spine of the book, although you would not need to put this information in a reference list

Photocopying from books and journals

Photocopying material from books or journals to read later may seem like a good idea (e.g. when you find material that you wish to use in your assignments), in that you can 'do it later'. Although this may have some benefits, for example if your time in the library is limited, however, you may be wasting both time and money. If you photocopy you still have to make notes from the material at a later date. Photocopying takes time and money: there may be a queue to use the machine, you may have to buy tokens and the cost will soon add up if you copy a large number of pages. Do not fall into the trap of thinking that just because you have photocopied material you have read it. It is often better to take notes and a full reference in the library and save your time and money. However, there are a few occasions when taking a photocopy is a good idea, such as when you find an article which is a review of a subject that contains a number of other references or when the book is a library reference copy which you cannot borrow.

Tip

When photocopying from a book, also photocopy the page at the front of the book with the publication details (see Fig. 3.1).

Most copying machines have a function mode which allows you to photo-copy two pages on one sheet. Although the text will be small it will save you a significant amount of money.

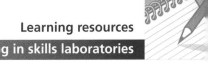

Copyright laws limit the amount of material that you are legally entitled to copy. Your library will usually have a guide on this issue or you can check with the librarian. Illustrations are subject to copyright laws in the same way as written material. Always take a full reference if you are copying a chart or diagram; this should be listed in your sources if you use this material in an essay or project.

Searching catalogues and databases

It is a good idea to start looking for information as soon as possible so that you become confident in finding your way around the library, which will be the main source of your information. You can either browse the shelves or look for material electronically through the library catalogue (all the material available in the library). The way the books are organised in sections upon the shelves will depend on the actual words in the title of a book which will place it in a specific category in the catalogue system. For example, a book with 'study skills' as the title may be in a completely different section from one entitled 'writing for health care professionals'. There will normally be guides to the system on the sides of the shelves.

Alternatively, you can use the computer-based catalogues to find information. Your librarian will be able to help. In addition, the library will run courses on using the specific databases available at your institution, which will help you search for a wide range of material from journals, some of which may be available in your university library. The library will have a list of the journals that it holds but you may have to try another library. Most universities take a range of journals related to the courses they run but if you want a copy of an article from another journal you may have to request material from another library for which there will be a fee. In addition, your university library is likely to subscribe to online journals which you can read and take notes from; however, if you want a paper copy, there is likely to be a charge.

LEARNING IN SKILLS LABORATORIES

The skills laboratory will have models, manikins and equipment to practise with and to help you link theory with nursing practice. Learning new psychomotor skills is always a challenge and it may be that you will find some practical skills difficult at first. The answer is to practise in the skills laboratory as it is difficult to do this on patients if you do not feel confident. Many universities have video/DVD materials and/or CD-ROMs to provide visual instruction. The best way to use these materials is in a small group. Watch the video, practise the skill and observe each other; then watch the video again and compare your performances. It is important to 'do' the skills rather than just read about them. Only by carrying out the skill will you know whether you can perform it correctly. In addition, you will find it easier to remember if you have actually done it.

Placement staff as learning resources

In practice placements there will be staff whose role is to help you learn. These are trained mentors, practice education facilitators and lecture practitioners. There will also be other resources such as reading materials. The Nursing and Midwifery Council (NMC 2004) requires all registered nurses to take responsibility for facilitating student learning in practice areas.

Mentors/assessors

You will be allocated a practice mentor who will be a learning resource. Your mentor will have been prepared for this role by undertaking a special training programme to be able to provide a positive learning environment for students. Your mentor will be a key person as a learning resource as they will support and guide your learning in practice.

Be prepared for your first meeting by having written your personal objectives in addition to those outcomes set as part of the course for the placement. Personal objectives are those you have set for yourself after analysing what you need to learn or the skills you feel you need to practise. You mentor will use these to help you develop a learning contract, which is a written agreement stating what you intend to learn and how this learning will be facilitated by your mentor (see p. 183). This does not have to be a lengthy document and usually one page is sufficient. The learning contract is underpinned by your commitment to learn and your mentor's obligations to help you achieve your learning outcomes or goals.

In this initial meeting the relevant learning opportunities of the placement will be discussed. Subsequently you should have regular meetings with your mentor during the placement, concluding with a final meeting to complete any necessary documentation. You should regard your mentor as a critical friend who will identify what you have done well and those areas where you should aim to improve in future. Having someone with whom to formally discuss your progress is an invaluable learning resource.

Study Tip

Working well with your mentor is important for your development:

- Be punctual and aim to maximise the time you have with your mentor – ask to change shifts to match those of your mentor if necessary.
- Engage with your mentor and be willing to help and enthusiastic to learn.
- Always carry a notebook to make a note of any questions to ask your mentor when you have an appropriate opportunity.
- If you feel that you are not sure how you are progressing on your placement, ask for a short meeting with your mentor for feedback on what you have achieved and where you still need to develop.
- If you have any issues about your allocated mentor, consult your placement guidelines or speak to the placement manager, link lecturer or your personal tutor. You should also consult your course handbook and placement guidelines.

Practice educators, lecturer practitioners and link lecturers

You will encounter other members of staff who will have a specific responsibility for student nurses while they are on placement.

- Practice educators (sometimes called practice education facilitators or managers) are usually employed by the health care trust and liaise with the university to provide overall coordination and support for students.
- Lecturer practitioners are employed to work in both the clinical area and as part-time lecturers on the university campus.
- Link lecturers who work full time in the university may have a designated link area where they visit on a regular basis to see students and liaise with staff. All these staff can help you by directing your learning while on placement and answering questions.

Asking questions on placement

The placement staff will expect you to have an enquiring attitude and you may have a lot of questions, especially on your first placement. However, when using staff as a learning resource you need to remember that the staff have a primary responsibility to the patients; it is important that you consider your timing when asking questions (Fig. 3.2).

Good times to ask questions:

- In feedback sessions with your mentor
- At report or handover times, or ward rounds (unless the area is busy)
- When away from patients direct hearing
- During activities that require less concentration, e.g. when making a bed

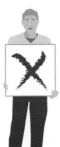

Bad times might be:

- When it would interrupt staff who are concentrating on performing aspects of care such as medicine rounds or treatments
- In front of patients or visitors

Figure 3.2 Good/bad times to ask questions

> **Tip**
>
> Asking questions is not the only way to learn. Make notes of your questions and look up some things for yourself. You are much more likely to remember and understand things if you discover the answers by yourself. Ask staff to clarify anything you do not understand.

Learning from other health care professionals

While on placement you will come into contact with a number of other health care professionals and you may be able to visit other departments where patients undergo investigations or treatments. These visits can be excellent learning experiences and you should aim to keep notes of each visit. Reflecting on the role of other professionals in providing care and working with other professions will help you to understand your patients' experiences.

If any health care professionals such as dietitians or social workers visit patients in your clinical placement, go with them when they talk to the patient and listen to the advice they give. If there is time, ask them about their role in the care of that patient. This information can be used for your portfolio and can also be a resource when completing essays as it will help you gain a greater understanding of health care. Professionals to look out for are physiotherapists, radiotherapists, radiographers, doctors, occupational therapists, dietitians, psychologists, pharmacists, social workers, speech therapists and specialist nurses, such as pain specialists.

> **Tip**
>
> Many clinical areas have pharmacists who are specifically allocated to that area. They are usually very happy to explain the different medicines that your patient is receiving. It is a good idea to start learning about medicines early in your programme so that by the end you have developed a good level of understanding. Because this is such an important part of the role of registered nurses, most university programmes require you to pass a clinical exam in administration of medicines.

Other learning resources in placement areas

You may find textbooks and specialist journals in placement areas and there will also be policy files and patient information leaflets. If you are unsure, ask your mentor to direct you to appropriate information. Senior students will also be able to help you. Make sure you always carry your notebook so that you can make the best use of reading materials on placement when there are quiet spells.

Learning from patients

Patients, especially those with long-term conditions, often know a great deal about their illness. The patient's perspective of how the condition affects them can provide you with useful information, making patients a very useful learning resource. Patients may be happy for you to learn from the care they are receiving but please remember that patients are entitled to refuse to be cared for by students (NMC 2004). Do not take it personally if a patient does not wish to be cared for by a student. Some patients may be emotionally distressed or anxious and may just want privacy or the reassurance of being cared for by a registered nurse.

When learning in placement – key points

- Always introduce yourself and make it clear that you are a student.
- Don't take it personally if a patient declines to allow you to provide care.
- If you make any notes about a patient as part of your learning experience, change names, personal details and places to ensure that confidentiality is maintained (NMC 2002a).
- Remember you must always be supervised when undertaking procedures involving patients until deemed competent to do so alone.

Peers – study groups

Although the need to learn independently will be emphasised, you will also be encouraged to work in teams and learn with and from your peers. This is important because nursing demands good teamwork skills and these can be developed through study groups. Resources can also be shared among friends. If you find a subject difficult, you may be surprised and reassured that you are not alone when you discover some of your peers are also finding it a problem area. Even if you don't think you would like to study in a group, you might like to join or start a study club or group so that you can benefit from shared learning. Some universities will help you organise such groups and provide space for you to meet.

SUMMARY OF KEY POINTS

- You need to develop skills of independent lifelong learning but there are lots of people to help you do this.
- It is worth spending time learning to use computers, databases and libraries as these will really help you throughout your career.
- Make learning easier by using available resources (e.g. librarian, personal tutor, mentor in placement) to make the best use of your study time.
- Use your personal tutor for advice and guidance.
- Get the most from placements by working with the staff who are there to support you during your experience in practice.

4

How to find information

Learning outcomes

This chapter will help you to learn how to:

- Get the most out of lectures and seminars
- Search for information in databases and on the internet
- Making effective notes from lectures, books, journals and practice
- Develop strategies to help get the most from your reading
- Analyse and critique what you have read.

The main function of universities and colleges is the creation of knowledge and its distribution to the wider community. Universities are vast repositories of information and as a student you will certainly want to use that information and may even contribute to that knowledge. Finding and using information is an important skill to learn and is vital if your practice is to be based on up-to-date evidence. It will also help you to learn and develop throughout your career.

Information is obtained from a wide variety of sources, including printed material, electronic media, practice experience, lectures, seminars and tutorials. This chapter will focus on gathering and using written information and learning from lecturers, tutors and colleagues.

LECTURES AND SEMINARS

Lectures and seminars are where the content of your course is outlined and made clear. The term 'outline' is important, because lecturers and tutors will provide only the skeleton of a subject; it is up to you to provide the rest. Lecturers and tutors will, through the lectures they deliver, try to provide you with a structure for their particular subject that will help you to understand and learn about nursing. Seminars are where topics and themes are developed and expanded upon. They provide an opportunity to review your level of understanding, and where you can challenge and change your thoughts through dialogue with others. Attendance at seminars and lectures is important; there is a strong correlation between attendance and passing education courses. The more you engage with your studies, the more successful you are likely to be (Pascarella & Terenzini 1991, Astin 1993).

The insight, behaviour and anecdotes of your lecturers and tutors at lecturers and seminars will help you gain insight into professional practice and what it is to be a registered nurse. Lectures and seminars are also where procedural information about your course is given; for example, changes to assessments, seminar rooms and important resources to use. If you are unable to attend, it is your responsibility to find the information.

Lectures are sometimes regarded as passive learning events (Ramsden 1992) where the lecturer's thoughts are transferred to the notepads of students without having to pass through their brains! The art of getting the most from your lecture is about remaining active and engaged: to listen, to concentrate and to think about how you make and form your notes (see p. 76). You will come across a range of good and bad lecturers; however, as a student, you need to learn from both. The learning is your responsibility.

Listening and concentration

A very important aspect of concentration starts before you go to a lecture, i.e. you need to decide why you are attending. Students attend lectures for a variety of reasons; for example, to learn, to be entertained, in case they miss something, because the lecturer is attractive, to socialise or because they cannot think of anything better to do. Although none of these reasons is mutually exclusive, the point is, that if you are not motivated to attend, you are unlikely to listen and to concentrate. If you do not have a good reason to listen to the speaker, you won't.

Preparing for lectures

Knowing you want to attend a lecture because you want to learn, understand and discover new things is part of your pre-lecture thinking. You also need to think about the subject or topic of the lecture. Even a small amount of preparation will help. For example, if your lecture is about the function of the heart, spend 10 minutes (perhaps during your journey to the lecture) reviewing the structure of the heart. If you do this you can then focus your learning on understanding how the heart functions because remembering its structure will make it that much easier.

When you enter the room or lecture theatre, sit where you can hear the speaker easily and other distractions are few; this will normally be in the middle of a room or at the front. There is usually plenty of space in the front row.

Active listening

You will need to put deliberate effort into listening and you will need to practise. Listening is an important skill for a nurse, and the lecture is a safe environment in which to practise. Active listening requires concentration: concentration is the act of dedicating most of one's effort to a particular activity.

The curse of concentration is distraction. Distractions can be external, such as noise, a change in lighting or a particularly attractive (or odd looking) lecturer, or internal, such as worries, dreams or thoughts of other activities.

Tip

One idea to help you concentrate is to make a concentration score sheet. On the score sheet keep a note of the number of times you are distracted. Students have found that the very act of keeping a score sheet helps them to concentrate (Pauk 1993). If you also record the type of distraction, you get a picture of the factors that disturb you, and you can use this information to take action to reduce such distractions.

If you are a good listener, you should be able to tell someone what they have just said to you. You should be able to recall what they said in your own words. Listening is therefore not just about hearing and remembering – it is also about hearing and thinking. The process of thinking about what was said will help you to remember the important issues.

Significant points and signal words

Try to listen to the main ideas or concepts in a lecture and note the facts that are used to support the speaker's arguments, summaries and conclusions. The lecturer will probably use important or signal words. For example, if lecturing about hospital acquired infections, the lecturer will probably use the term 'universal precautions'. This is a signal or key phrase and would indicate that there are a series of precautions that will fit under this heading. A lecturer is also likely to use small breaks or pauses between different topics; this may be preceded by a summary. If you are very lucky, you may even get a summary at the end of the lecture.

Try listening out for important phrases used by lecturers to emphasise significant points. As you become a more accomplished listener you will start to spot them on your own.

If the lecturer says something that you do not agree with, do not stop listening. Think what was said, and why you disagree; note the point and then, at a later stage, justify why you did not agree and go over the speaker's argument. Even if you agree with and understand what the speaker is saying, checking the points and the argument mentally during the lecture and on paper after will transform you from a passive listener to an active listener and learner. The term 'active listener' really means that not only are your ears detecting the sound but also your brain is thinking about what you are hearing. The most important aspect of the active listener is that they question what they hear and relate this to what they know. Box 4.1 outlines a series of questions that active listeners ask.

Box 4.1 Questions asked by active listeners

Questions about trying to connect with the way the lecturer is thinking:

- What is the structure?
- How is this session being put together?
- Where is it leading?
- How does it fit with what I know already?

Questions about content:

- What are the main ideas?
- What is the information that supports these ideas?
- What are the main keywords or important phrases?
- Am I finding answers to things I did not understand?
- Are the arguments logical?
- Are the conclusions valid?
- Is the material worth making notes on?

Questions focussed on you and what you want to gain from the lecture:

- Are there things in this lecture that I do not understand?
- What questions do I still have?
- How am I going to use the information from this lecture?
- What does the lecturer want me to do with the information (e.g. remember it, understand it, use it in practice)?

Adapted from Rowntree (1998).

Making notes

Making notes is an important aid to both concentration and listening, but you need to be sure that your note taking *contributes* to the main event and does not *become* the main event. It is more than likely that much of the material, particularly the factual material, covered in your lecture can be found elsewhere. Your lecture notes should therefore be brief, allowing you to focus on the lecture, but you must be prepared to make full notes when you can. Lecture notes are not the finished product; they should be seen as an aid to concentration and a basis for further study (see p. 77 for more information on note taking).

Asking questions

One way of enhancing concentration is to ask questions. Asking questions will help you to engage more with the lecturer. Make sure that your lecturer does not mind being interrupted. You can also ask questions if you have lost concentration. A simple request such as 'Would you mind going over that again?' will allow you to regain your train of thought. Your fellow students will also be grateful as they may also want refreshing.

FINDING TEXT-BASED INFORMATION

We live in a world that is rich in information and finding it is becoming easier and easier. There is a vast amount of information available, both in traditional written text and through computer-based sources such as the internet; all we have to do is think of strategies to get to and sort through information that will be useful.

Within universities and colleges a large amount of this information can be accessed through the services offered by libraries. Libraries used to be places were books were catalogued, stored and made available to readers. Today, however, libraries have evolved; they not only fill their traditional functions, but also serve as places where computer-based information can be accessed. Often these computer-based services can be used, via the internet, from computers at sites remote from the library, such as your own home, so nowadays you do not even need to be in the library to be using it. Despite the availability of information remotely, it is still a good idea to become familiar with your library. The library will hold a store of books that you will not have to pay to access and which are also free to borrow (as long as you take them back on time). Librarians will be able to direct you to books and appropriate sources of information, and will often provide training courses on how to use the library and its associated databases.

Databases

Databases are information storage devices that have a structure that allows the material contained within them to be searched and accessed. Bibliographic databases normally have stored within them information about the content of many thousands, if not hundreds of thousands, of articles. They can cover things such as

61

Table 4.1 The way in which bibliographic information is held in a database

Author(s)	Title	Subject	Date of publication	Type of publication
Gould, D.	Innovations in hand hygiene	Hygiene in health care	2000	Research journal

textbooks, research journals, trade journals, magazines, newspapers and even conference proceedings. Within bibliographic databases articles are listed under headings that help us search for the information. Common headings are subject, author, date of publication, title, type of publication and keywords. An article such as 'Innovations in hand hygiene' written by D. Gould and published in the *British Journal of Nursing* in the year 2000 may be stored in a database under the headings shown in Table 4.1.

The database is likely to contain more information than is displayed in Table 4.1; for example, it will probably contain a summary of the findings of the paper, keywords and exact publication details (e.g. volume of the journal and page numbers). It is important when searching to hold in your mind an idea of how the data are laid out within the database as this will help you to develop effective search strategies.

Computer-based databases have many advantages: not only do they offer easy access to large amounts of information but they are often also accessible from anywhere in the world, giving you the choice of where and when you wish to use them. In addition, they often provide a link to the original article if your library subscribes to that particular journal. You can usually email the results of searches to your personal email account.

It is still relatively unusual for a database to contain the full text of articles; more often they will contain a short summary, usually called an abstract. The abstract tells you in a few paragraphs what the article concerns and its conclusions. You can read the abstract and use this to decide if you then want to find the original article. You can often obtain online access to the complete article.

Access to databases

Most databases are now accessed via computer and, using the internet, many can be accessed from anywhere in the world. Some databases, such as the US Library of Congress, are open to all, whereas others have restricted access and are available to subscribers only. Fortunately, most universities and colleges subscribe to a wide variety of bibliographic databases and their students are granted access. Normally, the university controls access to the databases and you will need to be a registered user with your own password. The databases most commonly used by students of nursing are the British Nursing index, MEDLINE, Childata, PsycINFO and Cochrane Library (Table 4.2).

When searching for information, it is often worth looking beyond nursing databases; this is because different fields of study may look at the same topic from differing perspectives, and sometimes a different perspective can give us new

Table 4.2 Databases commonly available to nurses

Database	Description
BIDS	A service providing access to a range of databases such as Education and Social Science
British Nursing Index	Database that covers most popular English language nursing journals (strong focus on those published in UK)
Childata	Covers journals, books and reports relating to issues affecting children and young people; includes databases of children's organisations and news coverage of children
CINAHL	Cumulative Index to Nursing and Allied Health; virtually all appropriate English language journals are included
Cochrane Library	NHS electronic Library for Health; claims to be considered the 'best single source of reliable evidence about the effects of health care'
ISI Web of Science	Gives access to a searchable database covering a wide range of science-related journals
MEDLINE	US National Library of Medicine's bibliographic database of medicine, nursing, dentistry and allied health professions; covers 4600 journals, mostly English language
PsycINFO	Covers scholarly literature with respect to psychological, social, behavioural and health sciences
ZETOC	British Libraries electronic table of contents of approximately 20,000 research journals

insight. Examples of other useful databases are BIDS, ZETOC and ISI Web of Science (see Table 4.2).

Searching databases

Searches tend to fall into two main types: searches based on a topic or subject of interest and searches based on a particular author. It is also possible to perform searches based on the contents of a particular type of publication or even on a single journal title (e.g. *Nurse Education Today*). Subject-based searches commonly require you to provide a keyword for the search engine to look for within the article. A keyword is a word that encompasses the main theme or subject in which you are interested.

The power of computer-based databases is that they allow a great number of sources to be searched in a short space of time, and that the searches can be layered, i.e. searching for information on a particular subject, and restricting that search by another category such as year of publication. For example, if searching

Figure 4.1 Starting a search using ZETOC

for information on bipolar disorders you could restrict your search to articles published during the last 5 years.

The way to go about searching an individual database will depend on the database in question. Your university or college will provide you with the specifics concerning the databases that they support. It is not possible in this book to look at how individual databases allow searches to be constructed; instead we will discuss principles and give some useful tips and hints. Needless to say, some databases are easier to use than others and we would recommend, if you have access to it, trying the British Library database called ZETOC as it is a very user-friendly starting point (Fig. 4.1).

Search strategy and learning

When you search, consider how the information is likely to be stored (see Table 4.1). This can help you build a 'search strategy'. The art of searching for information is to find a way through to the information that is useful to you. Normally this means trying to find a method that does not provide too much information or too little. Searching for information can help you to focus your thoughts on what you are actually interested in. Before starting a search it may be worth considering the questions in Table 4.3. For each question we have given an example of the type of answer and the type of search that would be of use.

A strategy should summarise the way you are going to go about your search. You may start broad, and then narrow your search, or you may go for your specific area of interest. Using well-known authors as a focus for searches can be a good

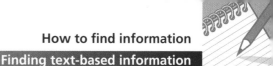

Table 4.3 Questions that can be used to develop a search strategy

Question	Example	Strategy
Are you looking for general information or something more specific?	Interested in general information on hand washing	Use search terms such as hand and washing combined, but also consider using other related terms such as hospital and hygiene
Do you want information from particular types of publication?	I just want research articles	Restrict search to articles found in journals only
Are you interested in specific groups of people?	I'm interested in hand washing, but only in relation to practice in the community	Use specific links (see Boolean operators, p. 67) such as: hand, washing, hygiene, community, practice
Do you want only current information or is date of publication not important?	I'm interested in the development of hand washing practice, so I want current and historical data	Use a search term such as 'hand washing'; do not restrict the search to a particular time span
Do you know the names of the important individuals in this subject area?	Dinah Gould has written quite a number of articles about hand washing	Use an author search using the name D. Gould in conjunction with a subject search using the term 'hand washing'

starting point, but doing a subject-based or keyword search may bring you a broader perspective.

Searching by author

Most bibliographic databases will allow you to search by author, and this is useful when you have some information about the key individuals working in a particular subject area. If author searching is supported by the database you are using, there will be somewhere on the computer page to enter the author's family name (surname) and the initials of their given (first) names (Fig. 4.2). Remember, with over 5 billion people in the world, many of whom share the same name, to be as specific as you can, and use initials of as many of the given names as you can. The database will indicate how you should enter the name; for example, in Figure 4.2, ZETOC requires surname and initials with no punctuation (Gould D). Take care to follow exactly the pattern (syntax) requested and place punctuation and spaces in the correct position. The most common problems people encounter when undertaking author searches are caused by not following the syntax or by spelling errors.

Searching by keyword

Searching by using a keyword or phase is probably the most common type of search you are likely to conduct. This type of search normally operates by looking

Figure 4.2 Using the author search function in the ZETOC database

for the word that you specify within the title of the article, the abstract or within the keywords specified by the author. Using as many keywords as you can think of will give you a wide perspective on the topic in which you are interested. Quite often at the bottom of the abstracts of research articles you will find that the author has listed keywords. Authors are asked to think of keywords that they consider represent the topic(s) of their article. Using these keywords can often help you locate similar articles.

Tip

Using keywords that will be found in many articles (e.g. 'nurse', 'nursing', 'patient') can result in a huge number of hits, many of which will not be useful to you. It is best to avoid using these terms unless absolutely necessary. If you do use them, combine them with other terms using Boolean operators (see p. 67).

You can ask most databases to search using all three approaches simultaneously (Fig. 4.3). When you search using a keyword, the more general a keyword the more articles (hits) you will find. You should therefore use keywords that are appropriate to the type of information you are seeking. For instance, if searching for information

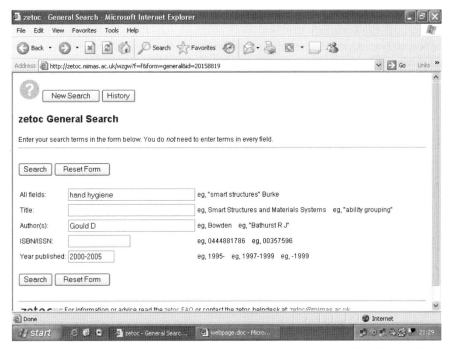

Figure 4.3 A search for articles by author (D Gould) using a keyword (hand hygiene) and restricted by date (between 2000 and 2005)

on hand washing, you will also want to look at work on hand hygiene. When using combinations of words such as 'hand hygiene' it is important to set up the search correctly so that you avoid getting articles with just the word hand or just the word hygiene (e.g. articles on kitchen hygiene). Using what are known as Boolean operators can help avoid such difficulties (see below).

Different words and expressions may be used to describe and discuss the same or similar phenomena. If you are interested in obesity, you may want to perform searches for 'obesity', 'overweight' and 'body mass index'. Similarly, searches concerning heart disease would be served using both the terms 'heart' and 'cardiac'. It is often worth using, as search terms, any abbreviations that may be used for the phenomenon of interest (e.g. HIV for human immunodeficiency virus). The more familiar you become with a particular topic, the more you will become aware of the terms and abbreviations that are commonly used.

Boolean operators

When searching by keyword it is not necessary to restrict yourself to single words; combinations of words and phrases can often be used. Many databases use what are called Boolean operators – simple instructions that come between keywords that you wish to use in combination. The three Boolean operators most commonly available are AND, OR and NOT. If you use the Boolean operator AND it tells the database that you wish to search for articles that contain the two keywords together.

For example the search term 'heart AND valve' would search only for articles that contained both the keywords heart and valve, although they do not necessarily have to appear next to each other. If you use the word OR between two search terms, the database will search for articles that contain either of your selected keywords, or both. Thus, using the AND operator restricts your search, whereas using the OR operator expands it. If you use the operator NOT, it restricts the database from including publications that use the excluded keyword. Thus the phrase 'heart NOT valve' would find articles that included the word heart but not the word valve. You can combine different Boolean operators; for example, 'heart AND valve NOT coronary'.

> ### Tip
> Ask your librarian for help with searching using Boolean operators. Librarians are very experienced and know lots of helpful tips and tricks.

Combining different search types

The real advantage of using a computer bibliographic database is that you can combine different headings. Thus it is possible to search for articles restricted by several headings; for example, by subject, author and date of publication (see Fig. 4.3). This ability allows you to refine searches so that you capture exactly the information that you require.

Search results

Search results usually appear as a numbered series of articles with the most recently published first in the list. By default, most databases will show the author(s) of each article along with the title of the article and in which medium it is published (book, journal, conference, etc.). In many databases, clicking on the article will bring up further information about that article, such as the abstract.

The search shown in Figure 4.3 produced a list of three articles (Fig. 4.4). For each article a list of authors is given along with the title of the article, the name of the publication that the article appears in and the details of where in the publication (volume, page numbers) the article occurs. Note that articles often have several authors and sometimes the author you are interested in will not be first in the author list for a particular article. In this database (ZETOC) it is possible to obtain an abstract of the article by clicking on the number on the left-hand side of the screen. Note that the way in which the results appear will vary depending on the database and you will need to become familiar with those that you use. If you get stuck, ask your librarian for help.

Using reviews and systematic reviews

Review articles are concerned with the discussion and summary of the important items of research and thinking on a particular topic. As well as being interesting to read, review articles can be very useful when conducting searches. Review articles

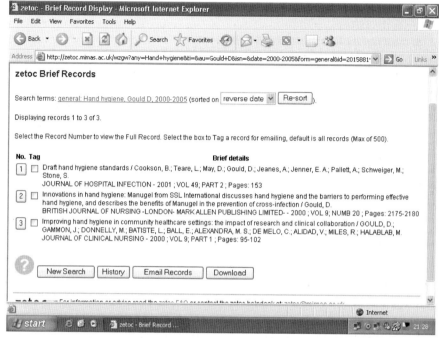

Figure 4.4 Results from the ZETOC search shown in Figure 4.3

will contain not only a summary of information from a range of articles, but also the references to those articles. The author of the review will usually have commented on and performed some analysis of individual articles. A review article is almost like a database with commentary. Some reviews are known as systematic reviews; this means that a strict criteria-based system has been used to dictate whether or not an article is considered within the review.

Thus, the articles within a systematic review would have been judged by the authors to meet certain described quality criteria. The most well-known systematic reviews in health are known as Cochrane Reviews (see www.nelh.nhs.uk/cochrane.asp).

Finding information on the internet

The internet is a network of interconnected computers that no one individual owns. The computers are connected electronically and they communicate with each other. Because many thousands, if not millions, of computers are attached to this network, the capacity of the system to store information is huge. You can normally access the internet via your university. The internet is often referred to as the 'web'. In order to access the internet from home, you will need a modem and an internet service provider (ISP). The ISP is normally an organisation that allows you to connect to a special computer called a server, which is linked (electronically) to the wider internet. When you use the internet at your university, the university is acting as the ISP.

At most universities the staff in the library will usually be the ones who teach you how to get the most from the internet. They will be able to show you how to access useful information on the internet and how to use the various search engines and databases.

Accessing the internet

To access the internet you need to have some software on the computer that you are using called a browser. There are two main browsers on the market: Microsoft Explorer® and Netscape Navigator®. They are similar to each other and at least one, and sometimes both, will be found on most PCs. Browsers read and translate internet files so that you can view them. They also allow you to move between internet files and pages with relative ease.

Hypertext links

Most internet pages are written in a special computer language called hypertext mark-up language (html) which allows internet pages and files to be linked to each other. The most common form of web pages use what are called hypertext links, links that connect you to other parts of the web page you are currently using or to other web pages. A hypertext link (text) tends to be highlighted on a page either by being underlined or distinguished by some other form of highlighting (e.g. blue writing). In addition, hypertext links can be images or figures. You can always tell when your cursor is on a hypertext link because the cursor symbol will change from an arrow to a pointing finger (Fig. 4.5).

Internet pages

Both Microsoft Explorer and Netscape Navigator have a similar layout. They have a navigation toolbar at the top and a dialogue box where you can write the address of web pages that you wish to visit (Fig. 4.6). The navigation toolbar has a series of buttons that help in managing your travel (sometimes called surfing) through the internet. If you know the name (address) of the site you wish to visit, type its details into the dialogue box and then press enter on your keyboard, or click on the 'Go' button next to the address box. The buttons on the navigation bar provide easy access to a range of functions, the most useful of which are outlined below.

Figure 4.6 shows an example from Microsoft Explorer; Netscape Navigator looks similar and has a similar navigation bar. Web pages are not all alike; the web page in Figure 4.5 is a page designed for the students of City University, London. Like most pages it has many hypertext links that will connect you with other pages, and those pages will have links to other pages. If you can imagine a series of pages all linked together, it is easy to see how the term 'web' came about. It is probably harder to imagine that all these pages can be accessed and linked both nationally and internationally. It is easy to become lost within the web, and this is where your 'Home' button comes in useful (see Fig. 4.6). The home button will take you back to the web page that your browser automatically starts with. This is the button above the address that has a little house on it.

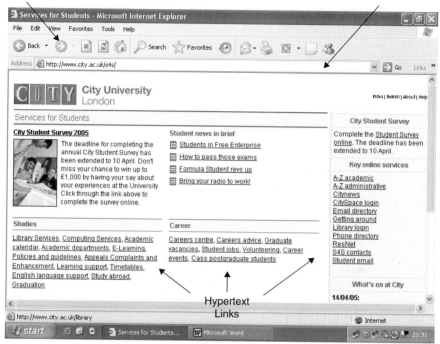

Figure 4.5 A web page showing the hypertext links

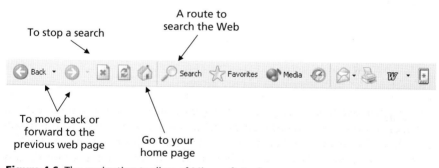

Figure 4.6 The navigation toolbar of Microsoft Explorer

Home page

Your university or college will usually set the home page. If you have your own computer you can choose a home page that suits your needs. Normally, when you first buy a computer the home page will be set by the manufacturer; however, you can change the home page yourself (or get a friend to). Explaining how to change the home page is beyond the scope of this book, but to find out, try using the built-in help function of the software, normally found at the top of the page. The manufacturer's (publisher's) guide to your current internet browser is usually helpful. A useful internet site is www.internet101.org.

Using an internet search engine

Searching the internet is bit like searching bibliographies, although the information on web pages is not sorted into any particular order and therefore the categories that you use are somewhat restricted. To search the internet, a device called a 'search engine' is used. These can usually be accessed from your home site. The most popular search engine is Google (www.google.co.uk); other well-known engines are Yahoo (www.yahoo.co.uk) and Ask Jeeves (www.ask.co.uk). Most search engines allow you to enter a keyword or phrase that the computer will search for across the internet. The search engine will then produce a list of web pages and sites containing your keyword. The exact mechanism used by search engines varies, so try using more than one.

Using keywords and phrases in search engines

As with bibliographic databases, using common words will tend to produce very long lists of results. Each website listed in the results is referred to as a hit. If, for example, you enter the word 'cardiac' in Google, over 4 million hits will be generated, and using the phrase 'care of the elderly' just 72,400. While even 72,400 may be excessive, search engines do rank the sites in order of 'perceived relevance'. The relevant information is usually within the first 0–50 sites.

In one of the above examples we used a single word and a phrase. In general, internet searches are made more specific by adding more words, because the search will be restricted to just those sites with all the words that you have used, in the same way as using the Boolean operator AND (see p. 67). Using a phrase and enclosing it in inverted commas (as we did with 'care of the elderly') restricts the search to just those sites using that exact phrase. Most search engines support the use of Boolean operators within their advanced facilities and some will let you confine your search to certain domains (see p. 73).

Unlike email systems, most search engines are not case sensitive, so searching for 'HOMEOSTASIS' or 'homeostasis' should get the same results. Some search engines allow you to browse through by subject category. This is, in fact, the basis of the commonly used search engine Yahoo and can also be carried out within Google's advanced options. Category-based searches are a good idea if you are not sure about which keyword to use. If you are interested in the mental health aspects of care of a patient with Parkinson's disease you may find it more fruitful to search for '*Parkinson's disease*' within the category *Mental Health*.

Internet and quality

Quality is an issue for the internet because anyone can post information to be retrieved by others, and it is relatively easy to give the impression that the material has come from a high quality source. Unlike books and journals, where often an editorial team has made a judgement on the quality and accuracy of the content, no such safeguard is in place for most information and material placed on the web (internet). Therefore, when using the web you are the person who must make the decision about the reliability and suitability of a particular article or web page. It is true that you also need to make decisions about other forms of information, but – unlike books, journals and magazines – it is often not clear from web pages who or what organisation has actually produced the material. Indeed, it is quite easy to find pages on the web where the organisation responsible for the material is deliberately trying to be obscure. Much web-based material is highly subjective (biased) and can be misleading, and in general should be treated with caution. Below, we have given some guidelines to help you make decisions about how accurate and impartial web-based material is likely to be.

Using web-based material

There is a clear difference between web pages and other types of material that are available via the web; for example, journal articles, government papers and documents can often be obtained via the web. This section concentrates on web pages, i.e. material that has been generated specifically to be used with the web.

When you find a web page that interests you, try to find out who the author is; an individual is less likely to put their name to work if it is incorrect. If there is a name attached to the site, are contact details available? Do the contact details work? If there is no name, but an organisation, are there contact details for that organisation? If an individual or organisation is willing to provide their name and contact details, it suggests that they are willing to take responsibility for putting the information on the internet and therefore they are likely to have good reason to believe the information to be true.

Type of site or domain

Sometimes you can tell the origin of a site from its address. An internet address is called a URL (universal resource locator). For example, City University's website address is http://www.city.ac.uk. The first part of the address tells computers what language the computer file is written in (http stands for hypertext transfer protocol). The next part of the address (www) stands for World Wide Web. This tells the computer what network the file page should be on; in this case the World Wide Web. The address indicates the server, or at least a name given to the server by the owner; in this example it is called 'City'. The server is followed by that part of the address which indicates the type of organisation the site belongs to (e.g. in the UK, 'ac' means academic) and finally (except for the USA) there is an indication of the country where the server is based. Taken together the part of the address *www.city.ac.uk* is known as the domain. In the example of our university's website, we know that we are dealing with a World Wide Web page owned by an organisation which has called its server 'City' and that it is an academic website based in the UK. Table 4.4 list some of the organisation codes in common use.

Each country except the USA has a country code; for example, uk (United Kingdom), ca (Canada), nz (New Zealand) and fr (France).

From the web address it is possible to get an indication of both the name of the organisation and its type. It is important to identify the organisation that is promoting the site as this will affect how impartial or biased the information is likely to be. You would not expect an anti-abortion site and a 'pro-choice' site to give you the same information in the same way. Websites may not be up-front about which side of an argument they stand on; caution is always required.

Table 4.4 Types of organisation code

Code	Site type
edu	Indicates educational establishments although not in UK
org	Indicates organisations such as charities and not-for-profit organisations
ac	Is used for further and higher education establishments in the UK
nhs	UK National Health Service organisations and trusts
co	Indicates a company normally based outside North America
com	Indicates a commercial company often based in North America
gov	Indicates government-linked sites
net	Indicates a network site

The country of origin can also have an impact on the information. In relation to health issues, different countries – as in most things – have differing cultures. In France, for example, the use of suppositories as a means to deliver drugs is common, but is less common in the UK.

Authority and websites

When thinking about authority, we consider what makes the individual believable and trustworthy, and whether they are likely to be a reliable source of information on the topic. For instance, the authors of this book have both been lecturers in universities for many years and have had experience working with students in higher education. In addition, this book has been through a review process. Taken together, these factors would give this book authority on the subject of study skills and higher education. What gives the web page you are reading the same authority? As you become more experienced at analysing and evaluating information, authority will become less important to you, because you will be able to evaluate the quality of the arguments for yourself. However, looking for authority is a good starting point.

As well as an individual's authority, we can look for an organisation's authority. Here, what we would be looking for is that we recognise and respect a particular organisation. For example, sites that are maintained by organisations such as the World Health Organization (WHO), the National Health Service (NHS) or professional bodies are likely to contain information that has been scrutinised for accuracy. Be suspicious about sites from organisations you are not familiar with and always consider what gives an organisation authority.

Content of the website

Having investigated the authority of the source, the next thing to look at is the content. Try considering these simple questions when assessing a web site:

- What has this web page been created for (e.g. to sell me something, to entertain, to persuade, to inform, to promote)?

> ## Box 4.2 Internet questions
>
> Think of a topic such as 'Passive smoking and lung cancer' and conduct an internet search using this term. Briefly, review the sites you have found, select three sites and evaluate each site using the ideas described in this section. Compare each site and identify similarities and differences. Score each site from 1 to 5 (5 = highest score) for each of the following attributes:
>
> - Authority
> - Ease of locating the source
> - Accuracy
> - Design

- Are there important things that it does not say (e.g. not mention side effects of a particular therapy)?
- Does the site express opinions? Is it ambiguous? Does it use emotional language?
- Are statements of facts supported by references to the source of that information?
- Are the sources accurate? (You will need to do some investigation.)
- How old is the site? (Just as information published in books becomes out of date, so does information published on the web.)

Next, check the information against similar sites. Information that is accurate may be repeated on other sites.

Construction of the website

The last clue to quality is the construction of the site. Does it work? Is the site organised well? Does it follow a logical path? Are any arguments constructed well? Do the hypertext links work? Is the site's use of English correct or does it contain spelling and grammatical errors? Try the exercise in Box 4.2. How did the sites you looked at compare? What criteria did you use to make your decisions?

It is good to treat all sources of information with healthy scepticism, but you need to treat internet pages with even more scepticism because, in general, there is less control on what gets onto the internet than into other text-based media. Remember, you are the ultimate judge of the quality of sources of information. Information on how to correctly reference material found on the web can be found in Chapter 6; later sections of this chapter will discuss how to make effective notes and learn from text-based material.

Information gathering from practice experience

Learning from practice experience has a long history and is linked to the general idea of experience-based learning. Although we learn in many ways, it is generally acknowledged that most of our understanding is derived from experience. We can learn from a whole variety of experiences, such as our social life, sporting activity, family life, voluntary activities, work and even holidays. One of the issues with expe-rience-based learning (experiential learning) is that it can be very inefficient and unpredictable. Sometimes we will have experiences that we do not learn from. A lot of our experiences (e.g. making toast) are learning experiences the first few times we do them, but not when we do them for the hundredth time. In order to make your learning from experience efficient, you need to (if the experience is planned) think about what you want to learn before an experience and reflect on what you did learn after the experience.

Experience-based learning can be either informal (i.e. not arranged or planned) or formal (planned and directed). Formal experiential learning should be designed to help you focus on learning from experience. It should include opportunities to plan what you are going to learn and how you are going to learn it. It should include periods of reflection and debriefing where you can 'unpick' exactly what you have learned. This is not to say that all your experiences in placements will be planned, and in fact many will not be. What is hoped is that the formal processes established to support learning will allow all the potential learning available to you in placement to be captured.

Experience-based learning is different from other forms of learning because the learning is gained through our senses and therefore, as our brains gather informa-tion, that information interacts with our emotions. The way in which we make sense of and understand that information belongs much more to ourselves (intrinsic) than to others (extrinsic). Experiential learning is, without doubt, central to health care education. Your experience will become vital in helping you to deter-mine the correct approach to care for your patients or clients (Hull et al 2005). To use your experience effectively, you need to develop the ways you learn from it (see Chapter 8).

NOTE MAKING AND TAKING

Rowntree (1998) makes the distinction between *making* and *taking* notes. Taking notes means being rather passive and done more to help us remember and con-centrate; making notes, on the other hand, is an active process, with the focus on organising information and thoughts. There is research evidence to suggest that students who make and use notes perform better at assessments than those who do not (Kulhavy & Dyer 1975, Annis & Davis 1978).

We make notes for a variety of reasons and take notes in a variety of circum-stances. There are three principal reasons why we take notes:

- To help us remember
- To help us learn
- As a formal record of interactions, events or conversations.

The form that notes take varies according to their purpose and our own particular style. As being able to make accurate notes will be an essential part of your pro-fessional life, it is a skill well worth developing.

Notes, when used in the context of study, are an interim measure between finding new information and learning it and/or using the information for a specific purpose.

Note taking in lectures and seminars

Most people will need to take notes during lectures and seminars, as they can help us to focus on what is being said. Later they will serve to help us remember and recall. Many lecturers will provide handouts of their lectures but, nevertheless, even if these are comprehensive, it is important to make additional notes; this is because research has shown that students remember more when they *make* and *use* notes (Kesselman-Turkel & Peterson 1982). When we take notes in lectures and seminars we are relatively passive; it is essentially a process of recording other people's ideas in a shorter, abbreviated form. Students often say they take notes during lectures because it helps them to concentrate; however, making notes can help you to become an active listener (Rowntree 1998) (see 'Note making and taking', p. 76).

> **Tip**
>
> When taking notes in lectures and seminars it is important to avoid writing so much that you learn nothing from what is being said.

You need to think about what you gain from a lecture that is difficult to find elsewhere. For instance, you will probably be able to obtain factual information relatively easily from textbooks. A good lecture will give you insight and understanding, and provide a structure that will help you organise your thoughts. It will also help you develop a sense of what the subject is about and how experts seek to understand its nature. You may want to focus your notes on these factors rather than on noting down factual information.

Perhaps one of the most often forgotten factors about lectures is that by turning up you are choosing to go to the lecture (see 'Listening and concentration', p. 58). Some reasons that students give for attending lectures are shown in Box 4.3. Does the box show any of your reasons?

> **Tip**
>
> Remember, the responsibility for gaining something from a lecture lies mostly with you. If you prepare well you should be able to gain something from a lecture or seminar regardless of how good or bad the presenter is. When you know *why* you are attending a lecture (see Box 4.3) you will be in a better position to focus on your learning and note taking.

Box 4.3 Reasons for attending lectures

The following are some of the reasons that students give for attending lectures:

To learn; to make sure I know what I need to (so that I can pass); because the lecturer is good; to be entertained (the lecturer is funny); because I feel I should; because my friends do.

Put these reasons in order, with the item that is most important for you first and the one that is least important last. Be honest: what does this tell you about your current motivation for study?

The Cornell system of note taking

If, when looking at your notes, you find they are of little use, they do not make sense or lack detail and structure, you need to think about how you take notes and consider the method that you use. There are several systems and strategies for producing notes but little research to show whether one method is superior to another. The Cornell system of note taking is really a system of preparation and review, and fits with several note-taking strategies.

The Cornell system (Pauk 1993) is a structure for note taking that can help people get the most out of lectures and to become better at learning through the process of note taking. The Cornell system uses paper that has been divided into two columns, with a box on the bottom of each page for reflection and review. The first column is headed the recall column, the second the record column (Fig. 4.7). The record column, which is used primarily for records during the lecture, should be wider than the first. The recall column is used for review, adding structure and reflection.

Preparing/using the record column

Before you go to the lecture, write what you have done to prepare for the lecture (in the record column); in the first column think about how your preparation could be improved. When you attend the lecture use the second column to record notes of the actual lecture. Use whatever form of notes you are happiest with and focus on ideas and explanations, and the examples that have been used to support them.

Reducing your notes

After the lecture, work on reducing your notes. Do this by asking yourself questions about the content of the lecture. Put these reduced recall notes in the first column. Reducing the notes in this way will help you to sort out the meaning within the notes and to make sense of them. It will force you to revisit the lecture you have just attended. This process of reducing your notes needs to be done as soon as possible after your lecture or seminar; this will help you to recall your learning from the lecture at a later date.

Recall column	Record column
Used for reviewing the lecture notes and writing short summaries. Helps with organising your thoughts	Used for recording ideas, explanations and examples using a suitable form of notes
Reflection and review	
Source of notes: e.g. Lecture on Research Ethics: 28/01/05: Dr. I. Knowit or Pauk, W (1993) How to study in college. Boston, Massachusetts: Houghton Miffin.	

Figure 4.7 A page from the Cornell note-taking system

Recite stage

The next step is to use what you have written in the recall column to go over what was said in the lecture. At this stage look only at the recall column, not the actual notes. This stage is known as the recite stage. If you are working with others (e.g. in a study group), it is a good idea for each of you to describe, using your recall column, what you think the lecture was about and what you think you learned. You may be surprised at the difference between your notes and those of your colleagues.

Reflection

Now that you are clear on what the session was about, you can start to reflect on the content:

- Was it true?
- How did it match with what you had previously learned?
- Was it logical?
- Did the examples support the argument?

- What are you going to do with the information that you have gained?
- What did your lecturer want you to do with the information?

This reflection is placed in the lower box (see Fig. 4.8).

Reviewing stage

The last stage is to revisit your notes periodically to review them. Reviewing your notes will help you to remember the content, but more importantly reviewing your notes allows you to add to them from your reading and to change them if your views and understanding change. An example of a completed Cornell note page is shown in Figure 4.8.

Notation style

The Cornell system is effective because it has a built-in process of recall. Research has shown that this is an important part of the learning process (e.g. Kesselman-Turkel & Peterson 1982, Kiewra 1987). The styles of notes vary but essentially they fall into one of three camps: linear prose, outline summaries or diagrammatic (Rowntree 1998). Most students start off using the prose approach but often find that they tend to write too much.

Prose

Prose-based notes are written in full sentences, with the temptation to try to write down everything that the lecturer says. This, however, will probably mean that you won't be an active listener. If you use this technique you must focus on essential elements and phrases and try to record the central themes, arguments and conclusions. The notes will be written in chronological order. This method can be made easier and more structured if you jot down a single sentence for each new point, issue or argument raised. Each sentence is given a new line and is numbered. This approach is particularly useful if the lecture is fast or not very structured. Leave space between points to add additional notes if the lecturer elaborates further.

Outlines

An outline will record the session in much less detail. Single words or short phrases will be used to capture the main features of the talk. The notes will tend to follow the session chronologically but this will depend largely on how the lecture is organised. Some outline styles use features to highlight more important points or to signify levels of complexity (Box 4.4). Although several different styles can be used, we will discuss only two: indentation and charting.

Indentation

Using the indentation method, general information is recorded at the left-hand side of the page, with more specific information placed progressively more to the right as it becomes more detailed (Box 4.5). Related items are retained together as a block of text with various indentations. The indentation technique relies on the lecturer being organised and delivering their lecture in a particular way (i.e. from the general to the specific) but not all lecturers work in this fashion.

Recall column	Record column
	Introduction to pain and its management
Aim is to reduce suffering	1. Pain management is about reducing the experience of pain
Why? – uncomfortable, distressing, also many consequences on rest of life	2. Pain can affect many aspects of a person's life. Examples: mobility, social activities, mood, confidence, ability to concentrate and how positive they feel. It can change relationships, affect sleep pattern and/or how much they enjoy life
	3. Pain is an unpleasant sensory and emotional experience associated with actual or potential tissue damage
We do not have a complete understanding, sometimes direct cause and effect. Gate theory useful	4. Contradicted by the gate control theory of pain see Melzak & Wall. Focuses on different pain states at the brain, rather than at the site where the brain perceives the pain to be. Pain is really a perception, and not an objective state of a body
Different types of pain occur, important division between acute and chronic Acute pain responds well to drugs (analgesics – what type of drugs are these?)	5. Pain can be either acute or chronic. Acute pain does not last long; it is short term and normally the pain and the cause of the pain are directly linked. It tends to be sharp but not always. Medicine-based treatments are very effective
	6. Chronic pain is longer term and often more diffuse, less sharp, not always linked strongly to source. Although not often sharp, it can be very debilitating
Chronic difficult to treat – alternative therapies	7. Chronic pain does not always respond well to medicines and habituation to drugs can occur; but addiction to opiate-based analgesia very rare. Alternative therapies (acupuncture, hypnotherapy, water) frequently found to be effective
	8. Chronic pain management often combines physical, emotional, intellectual, and social approaches to help the individual regain control of their life
Pain can be classified based on tissue of origin	9. Pain can also be classified based on tissue type, somatic, visceral and cutaneous; also neuropathic
Not really sure what was meant, is this linked to gate theory?	10. Chronic pain does not seem to have a reason
Reflection and review	
Pain is very important to patients. Sometimes it is difficult to know what to do for patients with chronic pain; many have "tried everything". Wide range of alternative to drugs available. Need to explore gate theory and clarify point 10. I'm not sure what use the classification of pain into tissue of origin is; does this help in the therapy, does pain from different tissues respond differently?	
Source of notes: Lecture notes from Miss Anthrope	

Figure 4.8 An example of a completed Cornell note page based on a lecture introducing the concept of pain

Charting

When using the charting method you need to have a good idea of the main themes that will be covered by the lecture or seminar. Many lecturers give an outline of the content of the lecture at the beginning, which can help when using this method.

Box 4.4 Example of the outline style of note taking

Pain management = −ve experience

Affects all aspects, e.g. mobility, socialising, mood, etc.

Unpleasant sensory and emotional

Gate theory = (Melzack and Wall) – look this up

Acute = short term

Chronic = longer, more diffuse, less sharp, but still debilitating

Analgesics do not always work; complementary therapies can be of use

Also emotional and social approaches

Classification of pain: somatic, visceral, cutaneous and neuropathic – look these up

Box 4.5 Example of the indentation method of note taking

Pain management – introduction

Management about reducing experience of pain
  Pain affects many aspects of individual's life
    Examples: mood, mobility, social activities

Pain is unpleasant sensory and emotional experience
  Caused by actual or potential damage to tissue but see also gate theory (Melzack & Wall)
  Pain is a perception, not an objective state

Pain can be chronic or acute
  Chronic is long term, acute is short term
  Acute pain – normally close link between pain and cause; with chronic not always the case
    Chronic pain less responsive to medicines, alternative therapies often found to be effective

You then divide your notepaper into columns that represent each of the themes (Fig. 4.9). As the session progresses, make notes in each column according to the theme being discussed. You will have quite narrow columns, so your note taking will be restricted to keywords and phrases, thus limiting the amount of writing required. This approach is useful for discussion and seminars; it will also help you to make connections between different ideas.

Diagrammatic

There are several different names given to diagrammatic note taking such as spray, spider and mind maps. The use of such diagrams requires active engagement with the lecture as the note taker is required to relate concepts, facts and examples to

Pain management – introduction		
Impacts	What pain is	Approaches to therapies
Wide ranging – physical, e.g. mobility, sleep patterns Emotional, e.g. confidence mood Social, e.g. altered relationships; inability to go out; also linked to other factors such as confidence	Unpleasant sensory and emotional experience associated with actual or potential tissue damage Contradicted by gate theory (Melzak & Wall), which looks at pain states of the brain Pain is a perception, not objective state of body Acute and chronic pain are recognised with different characteristics: acute = short term and site strongly associated with cause of pain; chronic can be more diffuse, not always linked to source	Management is about reducing the experience of pain Acute pain often responds to drugs, wide range of different types available Chronic pain does not always respond to drugs. Alternative therapies (e.g. acupuncture, hypnotherapy) often help

Figure 4.9 Example of the charting method of note taking

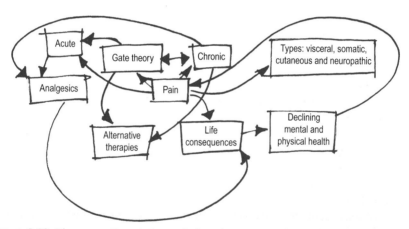

Figure 4.10 Diagrammatic notation style for a lecture introducing the concept of pain

each other. These diagrams tend to start off with a general issue, normally written in the centre of the page, with lines radiating from the centre for each major theme that is developed. Each branch from the centre is labelled. Sub-branches can be developed as issues become more specific or less important to the central theme (Fig. 4.10); each sub-branch is itself labelled. Some people like to use boxes for the themes and subthemes and then link these with lines where the various themes are connected. These diagrams are similar to those known as mind maps.

The advantage of a diagrammatic approach is that it provides a visual record of a lecture/seminar and as such is useful to those individuals who are visual learners (Dunn & Dunn 1978). The notes will also highlight the main issues of the session and the connections between the various points will be obvious.

The use of such diagrams is not to everyone's liking and will probably not suit you if you prefer to see information and ideas presented in a logical and progressive manner. Some people find that normal (A5) sized notepaper does not provide sufficient space and that the page becomes too full of information. A large notebook with double-page spreads may help. However, diagrams can provide a good base upon which to build more detailed notes, and can also be useful to use as a recall activity at the end of a lecture and for revision.

TAKING NOTES FROM WRITTEN MATERIAL

All of the above techniques can also be used when making notes from written material. Written material is, however, a very different learning resource from a lecture or seminar, and as such the way we engage with that resource may need to be adjusted.

SQ3R

SQ3R is a system that was developed to promote detailed active reading; however, it can also be seen as a system for studying (Robinson 1961). SQ3R stands for Survey, Question, Read, Recall and Review (Beard 1990). The acronym should be written as SQRRR, but is more often written as SQ3R. None of the stages is exclusive; for example, as you survey you will be reading and questioning – the focus of the next sections will be the difference between each of the stages. This system will help you to make good use of your study time because it supports reading for understanding. SQ3R has many similarities with the Cornell system, as both involve questioning, recalling and reviewing. You can develop confidence in using this technique by practising with a partner or within a study group (Fairbairn & Winch 1996). Using groups will allow you to exchange different impressions of your reading and, as with lectures, you will probably be surprised how different they are.

The SQ3R technique is most suited to making notes from your readings (notice how the language we are using has changed from referring to note taking to note making, the former suggesting a rather passive activity whereas the latter is a more active process – see 'Note making and taking', p. 76).

Survey

The survey stage is the part of the process that can take the most time because it involves asking not only the question 'What is this article/book about?' but also 'How is it structured?' and 'Which sections may be useful?' Surveying a book starts with the title, but you should move onto more informative sources of information such as the contents page or the index. The index lists the topics covered in the book in alphabetical order and details the pages on which each topic occurs. If you are looking for information on a specific topic, the index is a good place to start; using the index is more efficient than simply flipping through the book.

The introduction, the preface and the foreword normally contain general information about how a book is structured, for whom it is intended and, sometimes, the particular approach that will be taken. The introduction, for example, will often outline at which level of experience or expertise the book is written.

Questioning

Once you have started your survey and have begun to think about the significance of your findings to the phenomenon in which you are interested, you have entered the questioning stage of the SQ3R technique. At this stage in the process you will need to focus on the type of information and what you want it for. Useful questions are:

● Who is the article/book aimed at?
● Is the content evidence or opinion based?
● Is it new information or based on the interpretation of other people's work?
● What does the author think about this subject?
● What new technical terms are used?
● Can I make sense of what is being said?
● Is it written in a particular style?
● What questions am I trying to find the answers to?
● What am I trying to understand?

These questions should be based on your survey of the information and form the basis of your selection of the books and articles you are actually going to use.

Reading

In the question phase you will have been reading quickly to get an appreciation for the content of the material. In the reading phase you read with much greater depth and focus. In the survey stage you will probably skim read, in the questioning stage you might be looking in more detail at specific aspects (Payne & Whittaker 2000), but in the reading phase your approach will be more evaluative and focused (Fig. 4.11).

Deep reading is a skill that involves concentration, and Rowntree (1998) suggests that at this stage making notes should be avoided as this can distract you from the main task of reading and understanding what is written.

When you read deeply you need to be sceptical and ask questions of what is written. The aim of deep reading is to try to engage and be an active reader. When you read, know what you are trying to achieve and focus on what you are trying to find out and/or understand. The term 'deep' here is important because what you

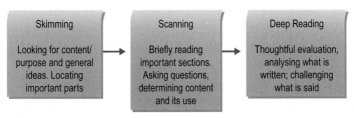

Figure 4.11 Reading for different purposes

want to avoid is reading at a surface level. If you read at a surface level you will fix-ate on trying to remember what you read rather than understanding.

> **Tip**
>
> Remembering is not the main point of reading, understanding is. If you understand what you are reading (e.g. why the pulse rate increases if the patient is bleeding), remembering becomes very much easier.

Reading in a questioning manner comes with practice. When reading, good start-ing questions are:

- Do I know this already?
- Is this information something I have never heard before?
- Is it of use and relevant to the question I am trying to address?

Asking these questions will help you focus your thoughts. As you start to evaluate the content you may ask some basic evaluative questions; these may initially be based on your current experiences and understanding of the subject:

- Does what I am reading match my experience?
- Do I agree with the author?
- Are there any contradictions in what is being said?
- Where have the facts come from?
- Are the facts right?

As you read you may also ask some more analytical questions:

- What are the ideas that support the author's arguments?
- Do the facts support the conclusion?
- Are the facts true but the conclusion wrong?
- Do the examples support the author? Are there other examples that do not?
- Is there an alternative conclusion?
- What happens to the idea/argument if some of the supporting facts are not true?
- How do the author's arguments/ideas accord with those of other writers?
- Are the arguments good, but others do not agree with them?

Finally, some questions focused on your needs:

- Is this author's work worth remembering?
- Should I make notes?
- Do I need to be aware of this article for an assessment?
- Should I discuss this work with my tutor, friend or study group?
- How does what the writer suggests relate to my practice? Will I change what I do?
- What have I learned from reading this article?

> **Tip**
>
> If you photocopy a journal article to read later, once you have read it, write on the back a brief summary of the main points and how useful you found the article to be. This will help you remember and also help later, if you return to the article.

Recall

Rowntree (1998) suggests that unless you make an active attempt to recall them, you are likely to forget about half of the ideas and concepts within what you read the moment you stop reading. The reading stage is best conducted without making notes; the recall stage is when you should make your notes. This note formation should be part of an active process of using what you have read. Using, as well as note making, could include discussing what you have read, putting what you have read into an assignment or trying to think about how you could use the information in practice.

Recall can occur during the reading stage. For example, you may just pause to think about and make sense of what you have read; you may put to one side what you have read and make some notes. Knowing that you will do some recall exercises will help you concentrate on what you are reading. The important aspect of recall is that you should make sense of what you have read without reading the original article. If you cannot recall and make sense of it then you must re-read. Recall can take time but is an essential part of the studying process and has been shown to improve success at college and university (Kiewra & Benton 1988).

The notes should be based on what you initially recall (remember) from your reading. The form of notes you use is entirely up to you. They need to be made in such a way that you can link the notes to the item that you are reading. You may, for example, give a Cornell note page (see Fig. 4.7) to each item that you read; each page can then be placed in a file under the particular subject or topic to which it relates.

It is essential that you record the source of your notes, including all the information that will be required to make a reference should you use that information in an assignment. Your notes need to be made in such a way that they are of use to you at a later stage. Mind maps and spider diagrams (see Fig 4.10) are useful at the initial recall stage but they will need to be developed and annotated if they are to be useful at a later date.

Review

The final stage is the review stage, which means going back over the notes you have made to make sure they are suitable for the reasons that you made them. In the review stage, check back to the original purpose of your study. Go back to the survey stage and ask yourself:

- What did I set out to achieve?
- What was the purpose of this period of study?
- Have I answered my questions from the survey stage?
- Do my notes make sense?

- What did I achieve?
- What have I learned from reading this article/book?
- Will I change what I do (e.g. the way I assess a patient's needs)?

> **Tip**
>
> Review your notes as your course progresses, checking that they still represent what you think about the subject. Update them as you discover new material and as new research emerges.

The SQ3R method is a structured approach to study. It should not be used too prescriptively, and can be adapted to the type of reading that you are doing. For instance, if you are reading about how to perform a well-defined and established procedure (e.g. giving an injection), you probably will not spend much time evaluating the content but more time questioning your understanding.

Although the SQ3R approach was originally devised for reading, it can be used in other circumstances such as lectures and seminars and even when you are learning in practice. You obviously need to think about how it can be adapted to a particular circumstance. In the lecture situation, preparation is similar to the survey stage and you could think of the type of questions you would like the lecturer to answer; active listening is akin to the reading stage of SQ3R. It is important to conduct the recall and review stages at the end of all lectures.

In practice situations, the survey stage is about preparation and finding out what a particular placement experience has to offer. The question stage means focusing on what you want to learn, the questions that you want answered and how you want to develop. In the practice situation doing/being involved in nursing activities is synonymous with the reading stage, but at the end of each practice day there is certainly a place for recall and review.

Filing and storing notes

Filing is the systematic arrangement and classification of the information contained in active files. Now that you have formed your notes, you need to organise and store them in some way so that you can find them quickly and easily. You will also need to organise any other useful information such as research articles that you have found. To do this you will need a filing system.

Storage

As well as filing you must consider storage. Some people may prefer to make their notes using a computer and store them electronically. Regardless of whether you make your notes using paper (hard copy) or a computer, your notes represent a substantial investment of both time and effort and should be treated as important and precious.

The main advantage of electronic systems is their portability and ease of access. You can, for example, carry all your notes on a computer disc or memory stick. If you own a laptop computer you can make and file your notes while you are in the library and update your notes as and when you find new information. If you do not have a laptop computer you will need to make paper-based notes and then transfer these notes to your electronic system. You will also need to use a separate system for any hard copies (e.g. research papers) that you want to keep for future reference.

In general, electronic records tend to be more vulnerable to damage and destruction than hard copy. This vulnerability can be overcome by making copies of your electronic notes. For example, you could keep notes both on a computer and as a back-up on a floppy disc or flash drive. Remember that, if you take this approach, the back-up should be stored in a separate location to the computer and that, as you change and update the main version, you also need to update the back-up version. Use electronic note storage if you are confident in your use of computers and file storage. If you are not confident, paper is probably the better option.

The advantages of paper-based notes are that they represent a tangible entity of your work, you have great flexibility over their structure and form, and they are easier to read than electronic notes. Paper-based notes also need to be treated with care. Use sturdy files that are not too bulky. We suggest using ring binders rather than wallet folders or box files. This is because with ring binders it is much easier to see and identify what is in a particular file. You can also buy small desktop filing cabinets – if you have the space, these are very useful.

Tip

When filing it is better to keep notes together using staples rather than paper clips. This avoids pages becoming detached from each other or other papers becoming lost if accidentally caught in the paper clips.

It is better to have several small files than one large file that strains your wrist every time you try to pick it up. In addition, should you lose a small file, it will be just a great annoyance rather than a complete disaster.

Filing systems

The principles of filing are the same whether you use electronic or hard copy. Filing systems should be designed to allow material to be easily stored and accessed. In any collection of notes you should be able to locate the item that you want without wasting valuable study time. This means that your notes need to be organised and filed in a manner that you understand and will not forget. There are three basic types of filing system: alphabetical, numerical and subject based.

- In alphabetical systems items are filed according to the originator's surname. There is a file for each letter of the alphabet. If, for example, you made notes on an article by John Smith, then your notes would be filed in the file marked S (i.e. S for Smith).
- In numerical systems each item is given a number and then an index is produced that locates each item.

- In subject-based systems the notes are filed under the appropriate subject. Notes on caring for patients with a broken arm might be placed in the Orthopaedics file.

With a subject-based filing system you will have to decide which collection of subjects to have and which collection of notes belongs in which file. Your subject files may thus depend on how you think about your subject. Within each subject file it is helpful to arrange the items alphabetically.

Subject-based filing systems are versatile and flexible. For instance, within subject files you can have subfiles. If you had a file called 'Cardiac', within that you may have subfiles (primary categories) for 'Acute care', 'Primary care' and 'Health promotion' (Fig. 4.12). You would then know that all the material you had collected pertaining to cardiac care was located in one place. If you were looking for an item on postoperative assessment of a cardiac patient, you would then look in your subfile named 'Acute care'. You can of course extend this so that you have subfiles (secondary categories) within the primary categories. Notes on smoking cessation clinics could for instance be filed in the main file 'Cardiac', in the primary category 'Health promotion', in a secondary category 'Smoking'.

If this seems rather complex, you may like to organise your files around how your course is taught. Most courses are now taught in modules or units. You can thus have a main file for each module and a subfile for subjects with those modules.

One of the problems of a subject-based system is that subject categories often overlap. In the previous example, for instance, smoking cigarettes is associated not only with cardiac health, but also with many other health disorders. To overcome this problem, items can be cross-referenced. To cross-reference, file the item in one category and place a cross-reference note in the other. This note tells you where

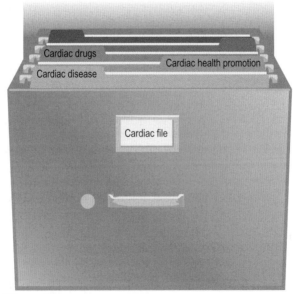

Figure 4.12 Filing system

the actual item is. Try to be consistent in deciding where to file items. Once a particular type of item (e.g. to do with smoking) is filed in a given file and category, it should always be filed there.

Sometimes items do not to fit into any main file subject area. At this point it is important to remember that the subjects you use to categorise your information are under your control. If you need a new one, make one.

Using a numerical system of filing can be useful for overcoming the problem of needing to file an item under a subject. In the numerical system each item is given a number and the item's subject and/or author recorded in an index. For example, for an item made of notes from Chapter 4 of *Essential Study Skills*, you would give the item a number, then record its subject, the authors (Ely & Scott) and its number in the index. Each item is then physically marked with its number and can then be placed in a store (ring binder or box).

The numerical system is not a very efficient system to use because of the problems of searching the index. However, this problem is overcome when the index is produced on a computer. Commonly available programmes such as Microsoft Excel or Microsoft Access can be used for this purpose. Within the programme, columns are allocated for the subject, the author(s) and the number of the item. If programmes such as these are used to form the index, you can create a file that can be searched by subject or author. From the programme you will be able to see the number of each article that relates to a particular subject; once you know the numbers you simply find the files in the appropriate box or ring binder.

Tip

While filing notes is important, you should not spend all your time filing rather than studying; make sure your filing system serves you and not the other way round. The earlier you start using a structured filing system, the easier it will be to do. Trying to reorganise badly filed material can be time consuming and irksome.

When you file, remember to file items that you are likely to use again during your course; your files should not simply be archives. Do not file something you are unlikely to use. Avoid filing copies of research or other articles if you have already made notes from them. Try not to photocopy too many articles that you have read. Use the library, make notes from the articles and file these (making sure you record the bibliographic details of the articles). If you haven't used an item for some time and you can't think when you will need it, throw it in your rubbish (recycling) bin.

NOTE MAKING WHEN ON PLACEMENT

Several of the systems for note taking described above are equally applicable to practice situations. When you are in practice you will encounter issues and experiences that you may wish to discuss at a later point in time. There will also be experiences that you want to remember so that you can use them for your own private reflection (see Chapter 8). In most practice situations there will also be some occasions where you will be expected to make notes (e.g. at 'hand over' on ward-based placements) and to use notes such as in case conferences. When recording notes in practice situations, you will probably need to adopt a style that is relatively rapid yet still provides sufficient detail to allow for recall. Carry a small notebook with you while working with patients/clients. Make notes of your questions and look up things for yourself rather than always relying on staff to answer your questions. Education theory suggests that you are much more likely to remember and understand phenomena if you are forced to discover the answers yourself (Entwistle 1997).

When you make notes at handover and in case meetings, remember patient confidentiality and do not use information that identifies an individual patient. Any notes with a patient's details *must* be destroyed immediately after use on that shift. Clinical areas now have shredders for this purpose. Information of a highly confidential nature should not be made on scraps of paper as they may be dropped and cause an inappropriate disclosure of patient details. Any written information about a patient, even in note form, may be used as a legal document.

There are a number of principles to observe when making notes during handover reports:

- Noting patient details – you should note patients' problems and proposed investigations and treatments.
- Using abbreviations – if you don't know what an abbreviation stands for, note it down and find some time to look it up. If it is more urgent, ask at an appropriate time. Don't use abbreviations if you don't know what they represent.
- Checking and confirming information – this should be done with the registered nurse or other health professional supervising at the end of the report.
- Preparing for handover – make notes of any questions you have concerning patients.

Tip

Keep an A to Z indexed notebook. Every time you come across a word or phrase you that do not understand, record it in your notebook. When you find out what it means, make a note of that too. Your notebook will turn into a valuable source of information.

ANALYSIS AND THINKING CRITICALLY

Being able to read text and decide whether the arguments are valid (true) is an important skill and one that you will be expected to do, as both a student and a professional. At university or college, the ability to analyse, evaluate and critique other people's ideas is often used as a means of assessment. Learning how to interpret and

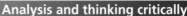

understand other people's writing is thus an important step to being able to engage with and complete such assignments.

Presenting an argument

When authors write, they are often trying to persuade you of something. It could be to persuade you of the benefits of a certain aspect of practice (e.g. hand cleaning) or to consider adopting a certain approach (e.g. to studying). Much of this type of academic writing is written in the form of what is known as an argument. Called a rational argument, this is not the same as one that occurs between individuals in dispute (non-rational); it should be a reasoned view or position based on conclusions formed from factual information.

The conclusion should be logical and follow from statements (premises) based on evidence; it is the use of empirical evidence that distinguishes a rational from a non-rational argument. Within rational arguments, you will also find statements that are designed to persuade or 'sell' a point of view. When putting forward an argument, e.g. 'Shall we go to the hospital canteen, the food is always good', we can be said to be trying to sell that argument (after all, some people may not hold the canteen food in such high regard). Some people are better at selling arguments than others; we call these people persuasive. As you investigate arguments you will find that what represents factual information is sometimes difficult to establish and on occasion we build our arguments on the best material we have that will support our position.

In order to decide what you think about an article, and whether you want to believe it and act on the information, you will need to confirm that the arguments presented are justified. You must judge whether the factual statements are true and if the conclusions drawn are correct. You must look for contradictions and discrepancies and for anything that does not seem logical. Look for the assumptions that underpin any arguments and make sure that these are reasonable; if an assumption is incorrect the argument will almost certainly be incorrect as well. For example, arguments for good hand hygiene are underpinned by the assumption that an important cause of the spread of pathogens is physical contact. When looking at arguments it is worth looking for potential alternative perspectives that can also explain the phenomenon or thing that is being investigated. Evaluating and analysing arguments is not always straightforward; it is a skill that improves with practice. The art of analysis is to pick out the facts and decide whether they are true, then look at the conclusions and see if the correct conclusion has been drawn.

An argument can be wrong or weak if:

- It is based on incorrect facts
- It is based only on opinion
- The facts are correct but the conclusion is wrong
- Important facts that would lead to a different conclusion are omitted
- There is more than one possible conclusion.

For a more extended discussion on the construction of arguments, see Part 3 of Fairbairn and Winch (1996).

Analysis

Arguments are not always presented in a straightforward manner. Look at the example below, and consider whether or not you think that this argument is valid. In other words, do you believe the factual information that has been supplied and that the correct conclusion has been drawn? (All of the citations are fictitious.)

> *Improving the hand hygiene practice of health care professionals is a quick and easy way of decreasing the number of hospital acquired infections (HAIs) that occur every year. Significant numbers of patients acquire infections during stays in hospital (Bloggs 2005). These HAIs cost the health services millions of pounds each year and cause an unnecessary burden on staff (Smith 2005). Tackling HAIs should be a priority for the health services, and it is therefore essential that increased effort be put into the hand hygiene education of health care professionals.*

Below we have numbered each sentence to help with the analysis. The first three sentences are premises, i.e. they are statements to support the argument. The last sentence (4) has two parts (separated by the word *and*). The first part of the sentence is an aspiration, a hope, a demand; it is therefore not a supporting statement. It could be a conclusion if it were a sentence on its own; however, read with the second half of the sentence, it is clearly an attempt to persuade us of the validity of the conclusion that is in the second half of sentence 4.

1. Improving the hand hygiene practice of health care professionals is a quick and easy way of decreasing the number of hospital acquired infections (HAIs) that occur every year.
2. Significant numbers of patients acquire infections during stays in hospital (Bloggs 2005).
3. These HAIs cost the health services millions of pounds each year and cause an unnecessary burden on staff (Smith 2005).
4. Tackling HAIs should be a priority for the health services, *and* it is therefore essential that increased effort be put into the hand hygiene education of health care professionals.

Having identified the components of the argument (analysed it) we now need to do some evaluation. Look at the supporting statements (sentences 1, 2 and 3): are they evidenced based? Sentences 2 and 3 have referenced sources and statement 3 follows from statement 2. If a significant number of patients get HAIs then it is bound to cost money to treat them and use staff time. In sentence 1 there is a claim that improving hand hygiene is 'quick and easy'. This statement has no reference and also does not seem to 'ring true'. Surely if improving hand hygiene were quick and easy it would have been done. We would evaluate this supporting statement as being weak and could even regard it as purely persuasive or even deceptive. When judging the conclusion (sentence 4) we need to make sure that this follows naturally from the premises. In this case, there is in fact only a limited connection between the premises and the conclusion. The conclusion contains the assumption that increasing the amount of hand hygiene education will result in better practice and that it should be a priority for the NHS. However, there is no information about the effectiveness of education in improving hand hygiene practice or that current hand hygiene practice is inadequate. The conclusion, based on the information supplied, is thus spurious, even though hand washing is clearly essential.

Do be aware that not all subject disciplines will agree on what constitutes evidence (Tapper 2004); what may seem a reasonable argument to a sociologist may seem a poor argument to a scientist.

Analysing an academic article or report

When you approach an article that you are going to read for the first time the following framework may help:

- What was the author's main purpose when writing this article?
- Are the assumptions realistic and evidence based?
- What evidence has been used to support the conclusion? Is the evidence good?
- What is the main conclusion? Is it reasonable? Is it based on the evidence that has been presented?
- Is there other work that supports the author's conclusions?
- Would I apply the findings to my practice? If not, why not – what are the doubts?

A useful exercise to help develop the skills of analysis and evaluation is to select a page of writing from a nursing journal and focus on identifying the various components. Read the article, then, using a coloured highlighter pen, identify the premises (statements of evidence to support an argument). Then, using a different coloured pen, identify the sentences that you think are there to persuade you. Finally, identify concluding statements, bearing in mind that these may be found not only at the end of articles but also after some supporting statements.

It is important to remember that, whatever your method, it is up to you to make a judgement on the quality and applicability of any particular article. Simply because a piece of writing has been published does not mean it is correct.

SUMMARY OF KEY POINTS

- Lectures and seminars provide valuable sources of information as long as you become an active listener and are able to concentrate.
- A concentration score sheet can help you recognise what distracts you from study and take action to reduce it.
- Computer databases provide easy access to huge amounts of information but you need to use the right words/items when searching.
- Librarians are expert at searching and well worth asking for help.
- Information on the internet (web pages) needs to be treated with caution and healthy scepticism.
- Note taking in lectures and seminars can help you remember what has been said.
- Note making is an active process that involves organisation and thought.
- There are a number of methods of note taking it and is worth experimenting to find one that suits you.
- Analysis and critical thinking are necessary when reading and thinking about other people's ideas.

5

Writing and presenting

Learning objectives

This chapter will help you to learn how to:

- Improve your written English skills
- Write clear sentences and paragraphs
- Understand the basics of grammar and punctuation
- Use your computer's spelling and grammar checker effectively
- Write in an academic style
- Write in a reflective style
- Improve your presentation skills.

This chapter will look at formal writing and presentations as a means of representing your ideas, thoughts and actions. Formal communication is a key life skill and a vital part of the life of a health professional. As a student you will need to be able to communicate what you have learned in a formal way. This chapter will help you to develop your writing and oral presentation skills.

WRITING

Being able to write competently is an important skill to have. It will allow you to write patient records with clarity and confidence. It will also help you present your ideas and demonstrate your knowledge throughout your career. Producing a well-written piece of work gives you a great sense of satisfaction; at university, well-written work will stand out. To be able to write competently you need to understand the basics. Practising will help you improve, as will reading more, particularly the work of high quality writers. Using study groups can help, especially if you read out your work to fellow students and friends.

Try the exercise in Box 5.1; you may be surprised how much we adjust the language of communication for different circumstances. For instance, when communicating by telephone we cannot see the body language of the other person or whether they are smiling or frowning. Communicating in writing is different from other forms of communication (Sully & Dallas 2005); for example, when reading you cannot see the writer's expression or ask them questions. It is therefore critical to remember that you do not write as you speak. In the following sections we will look at the basics of sentence construction followed by the use of paragraphs, spelling and punctuation. Students often ask whether grammar and spelling matter in written work; the answer is a definite yes!

Sentences

A sentence is a group of words that start with a capital letter and end in a full stop. The group of words, when read, must have meaning (make sense) without requiring or making reference to other words. Using writing to express thoughts and reasoning is necessary in academic writing. A well-written sentence should not leave you baffled or scratching your head to find its meaning.

Verbs and subjects

A sentence must have a verb and a subject. Verbs are often called 'action' or 'doing' words; they do something to the subject. The subject of the sentence is whatever the verb is acting on, not the topic of the sentence. The subject in a sentence usually

---

Box 5.1 The language of communication

List five differences between talking face to face and talking on the telephone.

comes before the verb except in questions. For example, in the sentence 'The man sat on the chair' the word 'man' is the subject and 'sat' is the verb. Typical subjects for sentences are nouns and pronouns. A noun is the name of something (e.g. dog, flat, person, John, family) while a pronoun is a word that can substitute for the noun (e.g. I, they, we, it; see p. 101).

If you can put the word 'to' in front of a word to form an action it is almost certainly a verb (e.g. to sit, to run, to swim, to speak, to learn, to write). The verb does not need to concern a physical action, it may equally concern a mental action (e.g. to desire, to ponder, to worry, to hate). Verbs are also used to describe phenomena or states of being (e.g. the verb 'to be', as in 'to be tall') or can be used to express possession (e.g. 'to have', as in 'to have a cold'). The verbs 'to be' and 'to have' are probably the most used verbs in the English language.

In the sentence 'The dog barked.' it is easy to spot the verb (barked) and the subject (dog). More complex sentences can have more than one verb and therefore more than one subject. For example, in the sentence 'Ian was good at running, except when Susan put stones in his trainers' there are two subjects and two verbs; can you spot them? (Ian and Susan = nouns; was and put = verbs.)

Understanding how to link verbs and subjects will help you to form understandable sentences. There are other types of words in sentences: the main ones are nouns (often the subject, e.g. *Peter* sat on the chair), adjectives, adverbs and pronouns (sometimes the subject, e.g. *He* sat on the chair). For more detail about the use of each, a good guide is Rose (2001) or Irving (2004a).

When writing sentences the most common mistakes students make are:

- To omit the subject that the verb is acting on. For example, 'work very hard' is not a sentence because there is no subject for the verb to act on. As such, it is unclear who or what is working very hard; it could, for example, say 'The students work very hard.'
- Not to have a working verb, i.e. a verb that is doing something to the subject. In the phrase 'I run to the emergency', the verb is present as the infinitive and as such it is not doing anything to the subject. By adding a working verb the sentence makes much more sense; 'I must run to the emergency.'
- Using the incorrect form of verbs. For instance, in the sentence, 'We was going to move the patient' the word *was* has been used incorrectly and should be 'We *were* going to move the patient'; both 'was' and 'were' are different forms of the verb 'to be'.

The mistakes outlined above tend to occur when we write as we speak. In a statement such as 'Observing the patients' the verb and the subject do not agree (while the patients are being observed they are not the ones *doing* the observing). The phrase could be transformed into a sentence by the addition of a subject, thus: 'We had been observing the patients.'

Regular and irregular verbs

Because they are familiar with English, most native speakers readily change between the different forms of verbs when speaking, but can make mistakes when writing. This issue can be particularly challenging for those whose first language is

---

Box 5.2 Regular and irregular verbs

Note how the verb 'to learn' changes in the sentences below:
- I learn by reflection.
- John learns in a different way.
- Today I learned how to measure temperature.

---

not English. The form of a verb is dependent on a number of factors, the most significant of which include:

- Whether you are referring to yourself, an object, another person or groups of other people (i.e. the subject of the sentence). For example, compare the form of the verb 'to have' in the sentences 'John has very little money.' and 'They have very little money.'
- The tense or time (e.g. past, future or present) to which the sentence is referring. Notice again how the verb 'to have' changes in the following sentences: 'I had lots of money.' and 'I have lots of money.' (Box 5.2).
- If the verb is referring to a continuous action such as thinking or running (here the letters *ing* are added to the verb).
- Whether the sentence is active or passive (see below).
- If the verb is a working verb or is present as an infinitive; when a verb is referred to by its name (e.g. to walk, to be, to have) it is known as the infinitive.

You will need to be aware of the appropriate form of each verb that you use for the circumstance in which you are using it. Some verbs do not follow a particular pattern, e.g. the verb 'to be'; such verbs are called irregular verbs. Rose (2001) provides further background. Irving (2004a) provides a framework for practising and further development.

Passive and active sentences

If you use a spelling and grammar checker on a computer you are likely to come across the term 'passive voice'. Using the passive voice is common in spoken English because it is less threatening than the active voice. In the passive voice something is being done to the subject; in the active, the subject is doing the action. For example:

> The manager agreed the amount of annual leave. (*Active*)
> The amount of annual leave was agreed by the management. (*Passive*)

In the first sentence it is quite clear that the management did the approving; in the second the manager seems to be doing less (it is more passive). The passive voice disguises the originator of ideas and concepts. For example, the sentence 'The book was written to help students study.' does not suggest ownership. It can be contrasted with 'We wrote this book to help students study.' In the latter sentence ownership of the writing is implied by the word 'we'.

> ### Tip
> Write down words that you hear in lectures in your notebook and then check their meaning and spelling when you write up your notes.

While there is nothing wrong with the passive voice, your writing can become snappier if you do not use it too often. However, academic, scientific and technical writing tends to use the passive voice to imply that the observers of phenomena took no part in determining the actual observations or their interpretation. It can also be useful when writing notes as it can avoid the need to keep using the word 'I'. For example, 'I measured the patient's blood pressure' becomes 'The patient's blood pressure was measured', and 'I noted the patient was becoming upset' becomes 'It became clear that the patient was becoming upset'.

Nouns and pronouns

As described above, the subject of a sentence is often a noun. Although the word noun refers to the word 'name', the term name is used very loosely. For example, it could refer to the name of an object (e.g. a hat) or it could refer to the name of a person (e.g. Joe Bloggs). Nouns can be things such as figureheads (the Queen, the Prime Minister), periods of time (minute, month, year), as well as things that are more abstract, e.g. heaven, beauty, happiness (such nouns are referred to as abstract nouns).

A sentence can contain more than one noun. For instance, in the sentence 'John gave an injection' there are clearly two nouns (John and injection). There is just one verb (to give) and one subject (John). The word injection is not a subject because the verb is not acting on it (see p. 98).

Pronouns are words that can be used to replace some nouns. For example, in conversation you refer to yourself using the pronoun 'I' rather than by your name.

Adjectives and adverbs

Adjectives and adverbs are words that modify, describe and enhance nouns and verbs. Sentences composed without adjectives or verbs would be fairly dull. The sentence 'The retired nurse sold a beautiful fob watch' contains the adjectives 'beautiful' and 'retired'. Without these words the sentence would be rather dull (The nurse sold a fob watch). Adjectives modify nouns and adverbs modify verbs. For example, in the sentence 'The nurse walked slowly' the word 'slowly' is modifying the verb 'to walk' – the adverb is telling us something about the way the walking was being done. Adverbs are easy to spot because they tend to end with the letters 'ly'.

However, there are some exceptions to this. For instance, if in the example we had said 'The nurse walked fast', in this case 'fast' is the adverb. Exceptions can also be found where the adverb is used to help form a question. In the sentence 'Why did the patient laugh', the adverb 'why' is modifying the verb 'to do' (expressed in the past tense as *did* in this sentence). Other similar adverbs are 'how', 'where' and 'when'.

Paragraphs

A paragraph is normally a collection of sentences that explain or describe a phenomenon, argument or point. Paragraphs are used to divide writing into discrete arguments, descriptions or points so that the information you are communicating to the reader is easier to take in. Paragraphs help to break up the text so that the reader is not confronted with a dense block of writing. There are no strict rules for the writing of paragraphs but remember that writing is about communication and paragraphs should be used to make communicating easier or clearer.

The length of paragraphs varies. It is probably a good idea to use relatively short paragraphs (three to eight sentences) if you are an inexperienced writer. A new paragraph should be started when you introduce a new point, argument or idea. The construction of a paragraph should be focused on the main point of the paragraph and support that point.

Often the main point of a paragraph is made by the first one or two sentences and the rest of the material supports, provides evidence and elaborates on those points. Look at the paragraph below.

> *Paracetamol is a widely used drug for the treatment of pain and the reduction of fever (antipyretic). It is now the most widely used pain relief in Britain. Paracetamol is used by health care professionals across the world. There are virtually no groups of people who should not take paracetamol, and interactions with other treatments are a rare problem.*

The first sentence forms the main point of the paragraph; the majority of the other sentences are supporting this point. The writer of this paragraph wants you to remember that paracetamol is a drug used to relieve pain and fever and that it is extremely widely used. The other sentences support this fact by saying it has global use. There is also an inference in the last sentence that its widespread use may be due to the fact that there are so few groups of people that cannot take the drug.

Paragraphs should be linked, i.e. the reader should not be confronted with a new issue in a new paragraph that they are not expecting. Thus a paragraph, as well as having a main point and its supporting statements, should also have a concluding sentence or link to the next paragraph.

In general, the supporting information should include evidence and comment. As you become more experienced you may also introduce contradiction or debate that is continued in the following paragraph. For example, we could have added a final sentence as below:

> *Paracetamol is a widely used drug for the treatment of pain and the reduction of fever (antipyretic). It is now the most widely used pain relief in Britain. Paracetamol is used by health care professionals across the world. There are virtually no groups of people who should not take paracetamol, and interactions with other treatments are a rare problem.* There have, however, been some issues with the use of paracetamol, particularly with its use as a means of suicide.

The addition of this last sentence introduces the reader to the idea that despite the widespread use of paracetamol, there are issues to be considered. The reader would thus not be surprised if the next paragraph expanded on the last point.

Sometimes a link can come from a following paragraph. For instance, in the paragraph concerning paracetamol, we could have omitted the last line and opened a new paragraph with a link.

> *Paracetamol is a widely used drug for the treatment of pain and the reduction of fever (antipyretic). It is now the most widely used pain relief in Britain. Paracetamol is used by health care professionals across the world. There are virtually no groups of people who should not take paracetamol, and interactions with other treatments are a rare problem.*

The widespread and easy availability of paracetamol has brought with it some issues, particularly with regard to its use as an aid to suicide.

The link between the two paragraphs is made because the new paragraph quite clearly refers to the salient issue from the previous paragraph. Other ways of linking paragraphs are discussed in Chapter 6.

Improving your written English

As indicated in the introduction, to improve your written English, the first thing to do is to increase your knowledge of basic English grammar. It is not necessary to be able to write perfect English, but what you write must make sense. As you increase your knowledge of grammar, you will become more self-aware of how you are writing.

Practise by giving yourself small writing tasks, such as writing short letters to your friends, or practise writing patient notes.

Read through your work as you write it; check each sentence after each paragraph that you have written. Do not leave checking your work to the end. Look to make sure the sentence has at least one active verb and a subject. Check that the verb and the subject agree (e.g. Many *people are* registered nurses) and that the verb form is appropriate to the tense (see p. 99).

Read the sentence out loud and ask yourself if it sounds as if it were spoken by a newsreader. Ask a friend who you think writes well (one prepared to be critical) to comment on your work. Practice makes perfect but practice works much better when you are getting it right. Another strategy is to do grammar exercises such as those recommended by Irving (2004a). These exercises should be built into your study time.

SPELLING

Being able to spell really helps. It will help you to write patient notes and other hand-written communications with confidence. This will improve the quality of those communications and thus enhance the quality of patient care.

Not being able to spell well is a common challenge (problem). The English language brings with it particular challenges and the proportion of people that cannot spell or suffer from dyslexia is relatively high among English-speaking nations. The high number of individuals who have difficulty spelling cannot simply be attributed to the quality of the education system. The problems with spelling in English probably emerge because the language is complex and has its roots in French, Anglo-Saxon and Norse. As Greene (1954) pointed out, three out of four words in the English language are not spelt phonetically, i.e. the spoken word sounds different from its spelling. Knowing that you are not alone may make you feel better, but it does not make you a better speller – that takes practice.

Before we look at how to improve your spelling we will briefly look at what is known about how we learn to spell. It is interesting to note that the ability to spell and the ability to read are skills that are not necessarily connected. Thus the ability to read well does not automatically mean you can spell well; it is also known that individuals who are aural learners tend to be poor at spelling (Riding & Rayner 1998). Spelling is a more complex language process than reading.

Spelling techniques

Spelling is a visual skill. If you misspell a word you often think 'that does not look right' or when asked how to spell a difficult word most people try to 'picture' the word or to write it down. For most of us, our brains must capture a mental image of a word when learning to spell it. So, if you want to improve your spelling, visual-based spelling study techniques (Frank et al 1987) are likely to be best.

Some spelling rules exist – for example, 'I before E except after C' – but these should not be used as your main technique as there are a large number of irregularities and discrepancies which mean they must be used with care. In the case of the 'I before E except after C' example, the rule, in fact, should be: 'I before E except after C and for words that rhyme with neigh'.

Using a dictionary

If you find spelling difficult, always work with a dictionary. It is better to check manually rather than use the computer's spell checker, as relying on the spell checker will make you lazy. The computer can be set up to highlight misspelt words. Try to work out the correct spelling for yourself or use your dictionary. The act of having to find the word or work it out will help you remember it in the future. Having read and corrected your work for the first time, repeat for a second time before handing it to a friend to do the same. Give your work a final read through, having made the corrections. If you use a computer for word processing, remember that even if your spelling is good, typing errors are common.

> **Tip**
>
> Computer spell checkers cannot identify when you spell a word correctly but use it incorrectly. For example, with words that have similar or the same pronunciation (e.g. there and their, except and accept) the computer often suggests the wrong one. It is therefore a good idea to look up the meanings of words if you need to check when and where they should be used.

Practising spelling

When you find you can't spell a word, you need to find out the correct way then practise that spelling. Carry a notebook with you and note down words that you cannot spell correctly and those about which you are unsure. In clinical placements, carry a small nursing dictionary with you and use it to look up technical words that you find difficult to spell. You can also use the dictionary to help you follow the technical terms that are used in your clinical area. When you have time, review and practise spelling the words in your notebook.

When practising, don't work on too many words at once; restrict yourself to three or four words per 20-minute session. Remember that spelling is a visual memory skill, so you will need to look at the correct spelling of each word, memorise it and then spell the word without reference to a dictionary. It often helps to copy out the correct spelling several times before trying without actually looking at the word. As your ability improves you will be able to memorise several words at once.

Practising using the words that you find difficult in short sentences, as well as writing paragraphs using several of your 'difficult words', may help.

Spelling by association

Another technique to consider is using associations. Using associations is a way of improving your memory and it can help you to remember how to spell words. For instance, when spelling the word 'grammar' it is *ar* at the end, not *er* like hammer and stammer. To remember this you might associate the word grandma with grammar; by doing this you will remember that grammar has an *a* at the end not an *e*. Associations may seem a bit odd, but if they work for you, use them.

Crosswords

Making little crosswords can help you to remember how to spell the words that you keep getting wrong. For example, if you have difficulty with the words 'precise' and 'exercise', placing them in a crossword will help you remember the form of the words.

```
                    E
                    x
                    e
                    r
        P r e c i s e
                    i
                    s
                    e
```

This method is successful because it helps you to remember the shape of the words.

Rhymes

Some people use rhymes to help them with difficult words. For example, to help remember how to spell the word diarrhoea: *Diarrhoea Is A Really Rotten Horrible Obnoxious Enteral Affliction.* Each letter of the word to be spelt is included in the rhyme and it is even better if the rhyme has some meaning – enteral means to do with the intestine and so is quite apt here.

Incorporating spelling exercises into your study can really help. Try using spelling exercises to improve your general ability. There are books that contain spelling exercises that can help you with this (e.g. Chisholm 2004).

Tip

Carry a notebook with you during lectures and tutorials and make a note of any words that you do not understand. Look them up as soon as possible and write their meaning in your notebook. The act of writing it down will help you to remember; however, if you can't remember you can look in your notebook.

Using the computer's spelling and grammar checker

Most computer word processing packages come with a spelling and grammar checker. In Microsoft Word you will find it in the Tools menu. Once you activate this function it will search through your document for errors. Make sure that your computer is set to the version of English that you wish to use – when you buy a computer it is often set to US English. If it is set to the wrong English you will either need to be able to spot the 'wrong' spellings or change the computer's settings (ask a friend or the university's technical staff for help if you are unsure).

When the spell checker finds a word that is spelt incorrectly (it checks words against its own dictionary held in the computer's memory) it will suggest words that are similar to the word it believes to be wrong (Fig. 5.1). It is important to remember that the computer really does not know which word you were trying to spell – it is just making a prediction based on what you have written. This means that the computer can get it wrong; it can select the wrong word, so take care. In the example in Figure 5.1, the word we were after was 'mistake' but the computer's first suggestion was 'misname'. If the computer comes up with more than one suggestion, be careful: read each suggestion, click on the appropriate word and then choose <u>C</u>hange from the buttons on the right. The computer will insert the word you have selected. If you are unable to select the correct word this may be a sign that you need more help with your ability to spell. The computer will not have knowledge of specialist nursing terms; you will need to look these up in your dictionary, perhaps then adding them to the computer's dictionary once you have confirmed their correct spelling (see below).

You can use the spell checker to improve your spelling by carefully noting words that you consistently spell incorrectly. Add these words to your notebook and develop strategies to help you spell them correctly (see rhymes and associations, p. 105). The computer will not be able to spot where you have missed out words or where you have spelt a word correctly but have used it incorrectly. For instance, the words *were* and *where* are often confused. The grammar checker will sometimes

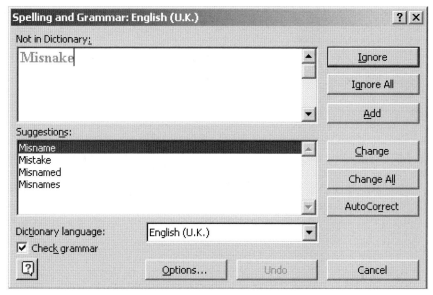

Figure 5.1 Microsoft Word's spell checker dialogue box

alert you to commonly confused words such as *there* and *their* but not always. The spell checker is not a substitute to thoroughly reading through your work.

Adding to the computer's dictionary

Spell checkers work from the dictionary stored within the computer. Often technical words that are spelt correctly will be indicated as misspelt words. It is possible to add new words to your computer's dictionary by clicking on Add – but make sure you are absolutely confident that you have spelt the word correctly.

Beware of AutoCorrect

Do not select AutoCorrect, which is a facility available on many spell checkers. If you do this, the computer will check every word in your document and when it finds a word misspelt it will always select its first option and replace your word. This can produce some amusing results but will not show you in good light.

Grammar check

The spelling and grammar checker can also detect errors such as when extra spaces occur between words, where words have been accidentally duplicated and incorrect grammar usage. Commonly, grammar checkers will indicate such things as where passive sentences have been used, where sentences are too long, where jargon has been used, where there are errors in punctuation and, in some situations, where the subject does not match the verb. Some grammar checkers will also suggest ways of rephrasing sentences and indicate if plurals have been used incorrectly. You need to use your own judgement as to whether or not to accept what the computer suggests;

with some checkers you can ask it to provide an explanation for its suggestion. If the computer suggests that one of your sentences is too long, it probably is!

PUNCTUATION

Punctuation was originally invented as a means of telling Actors of Ancient Greece which words to emphasise and where to pause when they were reading text. Punctuation developed further because, once most people could read, there was less need for reading aloud and more need to make sure what was being read was understood. In other words, as the written word took over from the spoken word as a means of conveying information, there was a greater need for writers to make sure they were understood, and this is where punctuation really helps. Punctuation is still there, of course, to help with the flow of the text and to tell us which words should be emphasised (Truss 2003).

To illustrate this, look at the statements in Box 5.3. Although they contain the same words, do the sentences have the same meaning?

As you can see from Box 5.3, punctuation is important and is worth consideration because it can change the meaning of the words that we write. When writing an academic essay or in clinical situations it is important to make sure that there is no room to misinterpret what you are saying; what you write must be unambiguous. When trying to write unambiguously, it is best to use short sentences. However, as we have seen above, even with short sentences it is not always possible to be unambiguous, so you will need punctuation. In addition, you will always need punctuation to indicate when you start (the capital letter) and when you finish (the full stop) your sentences.

Punctuation does have rules, but it is also rather subjective, and is subject to the whims of fashion; thus there is some room for interpretation. However, this room for manoeuvre does not mean that you can liberally scatter punctuation everywhere, or not use it at all. Punctuation is there to enhance our ability to communicate and to make reading more enjoyable.

The capital letter

The capital letter is quite straightforward: it is used at the start of sentences, for proper nouns, for the start of abbreviations and for acronyms (see below). Capital letters are also used for the start of part sentences (fragments) such as those you

---

Box 5.3 Punctuation

Cowboys are a central American concept.
Cowboys are a Central American concept.
and the sentences:
A woman: without her man, is nothing.
A woman: without her, man is nothing.

find forming the headings of subsections of books. When you quote someone else's work, if you are quoting the whole of a sentence the quote should start with a capital; however, if you are quoting part of a sentence then no capital should be used. As you will see below, quotation marks must be used if quoting some-one else's work and the full stop at the end of the sentence should be included within the quotation marks. For instance, 'It is an old maxim of mine that when you have excluded the impossible, whatever remains, however improbable, must be the truth.' is a quote from Arthur Conan Doyle's Sherlock Holmes (Conan Doyle 1892).

As with most communication, the way it is done and the rules that govern it change over time. In older texts all significant nouns began with a capital letter; nowadays, however, there is a general reduction in this. The key, as with all punc-tuation, is that you should always use a capital where it improves the meaning, but you should know why you are using it. In the example in Box 5.3 – 'Cowboys are a central American concept.' – without an appropriate capital this sentence is ambiguous as we do not know if the author is saying that cowboys are a concept from Central America or whether they are a phenomenon that is very important (central to) to American society.

Proper nouns

Capital letters are also used at the start of what are called proper nouns, i.e. the names or titles of an individual person, an individual place, an individual institu-tion or an individual event. Individual here means there is one of them and no other (i.e. unique). An example of a proper noun is your name. My name is Ian and when written it has a capital letter. It has a capital letter because I am referring to an individual (me). As well as names, identified individual positions should have capitals (e.g. Lord Advocate). The important point is that the individual must be a specific identifiable individual. Look at the two sentences below; can you see why the words 'member of parliament' have been treated differently?

Today I am going to see the Member of Parliament for Basingstoke.
I think that every member of parliament should take a big wage cut.

The first sentence refers to a single unique individual, the MP for Basingstoke, whereas the second refers to all members of parliament.

Place names

When referring to an individual place (e.g. Basingstoke) it should have a capital letter; again the general rule is that it should be an identifiable and unique place. As such, continents, countries, cities, towns and villages should all have capital letters. The same also applies to institutions such as Lloyds of London, Oxford University and The British Library.

Stemming from place names, we also find that words which link something or someone with a place are capitalised; thus words like French, German and Zimbabwean are given a capital, as well as words that indicate a person's origin or ethnicity, e.g. Afro-Caribbean. If, however, the name of the place is really only

---

Box 5.4 Capitalisation

Test your knowledge of capitalisation by correcting the following sentences:

1. The Hospital that I work for is called Greenwing.
2. my children are studying French, english and Maths.
3. I'd like an American muffin please.
4. My favourite book is Wind In The Willows.
5. The patient said, 'will I be able to go home today?'

Answers

1. The hospital that I work for is called Greenwing.
2. My children are studying French, English and maths.
3. I'd like an american muffin please.
4. My favourite book is *Wind in the Willows*.
5. The patient said, 'Will I be able to go home today?'

---

being used to signify a type or form of something, then it is not given a capital (Box 5.4). Thus 'french windows' and 'danish pastries' are not capitalised although your computer spell checker may suggest that they should be!

Some oddities

There are also some proper nouns that do not follow the rules:

- Calendar months and days of the week are normally capitalized, but seasons of the year seldom are.
- Words associated with religions are normally given capitals. This includes gods, festivals, periods, individuals and ceremonies, e.g. God, Buddha, Ramadan, Easter, Mohammed and Saint Joseph.
- The word 'I' is always a capital.
- When books titles are written, quite often each significant word in the title starts with a capital letter, e.g. *The Lord of the Rings*; however, the words 'of' and 'the' are not seen as significant and so are not capitalised. Another convention is that when the title of a book is used it should be written in italics.
- Abbreviations often start with a capital, e.g. Mr (Mister), but not always – for example, the abbreviation 'etc.' (etcetera). Unfortunately, you just need to become familiar with what is normal usage.

Acronyms

Acronyms are words made (usually) from the first letter of each word in the title of an organisation or an object, of which there are probably several hundred thousand in existence, e.g. the National Health Service (NHS), body mass index (BMI). In the past the letters making up the acronym were separated by full stops, but this is now relatively uncommon.

> **Tip**
>
> If using an acronym in an assignment, you need to write it in full the first time you use it and include the acronym in parentheses (brackets) after it; for example, blood pressure (BP). From then onwards it is acceptable to use the acronym only.

Full stops

The main use of the full stop is at the end of the sentence. A full stop is also used to indicate the use of an abbreviation and in websites and email addresses. When used in a website the mark tends to be referred to as a dot. For example, the website for the popular search engine Google would be said as 'www dot google dot com'.

Commas

The comma is probably where punctuation rules start to get less clear, and the guidelines that govern the use of commas tend to be flouted or ignored rather widely. Our advice is, use the comma to help the reader understand, and also to help your writing flow better. Commas have a number of uses, as follows.

Commas and lists

If you are writing a list of items they should be separated by commas apart from the last two items in the list; these are normally separated by the word *and* (or sometimes *or*). For example, 'In hospitals you will find nurses, doctors, physiotherapist, cleaners, patients and lots more besides.' Here what the comma is actually doing is taking the place of the word *and*. Consider another example: 'Depending on its severity you can treat a laceration with stitches, a plaster, just a bandage or you may choose to let the injury heal itself.' Here the comma is taking the place of the word *or*.

Commas before quotations

This is a common use of the comma, and its placement before the word 'said' allows you to pause before taking in the quotation. For instance, The Prime Minister said, 'Investment in the health service has never been higher.'

Commas and conjunctions

Commas should be used when writing sentences that are really (or as good as) two sentences joined by another word. For example:

> *The patient's family demanded that Jane should be admitted to hospital, as she was suffering from the symptoms of malaria.*

The sentence above is essentially two sentences (see p. 98) joined by the word *as* (known as a conjunction). A comma is used to separate the two clauses. Common joining words (conjunctions) are *and, as, while, but, or, because* and *so*.

Commas can also be used like parentheses in sentences where part of the sentence is there as additional information. It is there to give the sentence more interest; however, if it is removed, the sentence would retain its meaning. In such sentences the additional information should be enclosed in commas. For example:

Mrs. Stephens, who was 5 months pregnant, worked as a financial adviser.
Illness, although unwelcome, sometimes brings out the best in people.

The rule is quite simple; if the meaning of the sentence does not change if the section is removed then it should be enclosed in commas. If your additional clause comes at the end of a sentence rather than in the middle, the role of the closing comma is taken on by the full stop. Similarly, if the additional clause is at the start of a section then the role of the comma is taken on by the full stop of the previous sentence. For example:

When the phone rang, John was preparing to give Mr Jones a bed bath.
Sarah threw away the mop, which was old and dirty.

Now try the exercises in Box 5.5.

Apostrophes

The apostrophe is used to indicate possession and missing letters. As misuse of the apostrophe will annoy some of your tutors, think carefully before you write! There are several uses of the apostrophe but most confusion seems to centre on its use to imply possession and its use to indicate a missing letter. Apostrophes are not used to indicate plurals; this is where they are most commonly misused.

Apostrophes to indicate possession

Possession means ownership and, of course, to have ownership you need two things: someone or something doing the owning and something that is being

---

Box 5.5 Commas

Test your knowledge of commas by correcting the following sentences:

1. For lunch the patient was offered the following foods, soup, sausages, potatoes, carrots, and, bananas.
2. Working in the community is hard as you need to travel a great deal.
3. The consultant, who was very tall dominated the ward round.
4. Normally when I study I have some music playing.

Answers

1. For lunch the patient was offered the following foods, soup, sausages, potatoes, carrots and bananas.
2. Working in the community is hard, as you need to travel a great deal.
3. The consultant, who was very tall, dominated the ward round.
4. Normally, when I study I have some music playing.

owned. For example, in the statement 'That is John's house' the apostrophe before the s indicates that the house is possessed by John.

When more than one person or thing does the owning, the apostrophe comes after the s that indicates a plural, e.g. the students' bookshop. The position is important because if we wrote 'the student's bookshop' it would imply that one particular student owned the bookshop. Note that ownership here can also mean 'designed for', e.g. nurses' accommodation.

Apostrophes to indicate missing letters

Apostrophes are also used in what are called contractions. A contraction means that an apostrophe is used in place of one or more letters. Examples of common contractions are: *it's* (it is), *who's* (who is), *can't* (cannot), *I'd* (I would) and *they're* (they are). The biggest source of confusion comes from the contraction *it's* because the word 'its' also implies possession. For instance, in the statement 'The cat sharpened its claws' the word 'its' is implying ownership and used in this way there is no apostrophe; only when it is used to indicate a missing letter (as in 'it is') is an apostrophe used.

There are a numbers of words that imply ownership, such as *my, your, theirs, his, hers* and *ours*. 'Its' does not require an apostrophe when used to indicate ownership. But does when indicating a missing letter (it is), as in: 'It's good to be home again.' (To test your knowledge of apostrophes, try the exercises in Box 5.6.)

For more on punctuation, read the *Punctuation Repair Kit* (VanDyck 1996) and *Eats, Shoots and Leaves* (Truss 2003). *Improve your Punctuation* (Irving 2004) provides plenty of exercises, tests and puzzles.

Box 5.6 Apostrophes

Test your knowledge of apostrophes by correcting the following sentences:

1. I'd like some carrot's and banana's please.
2. It's the student's book festival.
3. Nurse's this way only.
4. Caring for people, its a way of life.

Answers

1. I'd like some carrots and bananas please.
2. It's the students' book festival.
3. Nurses this way only.
4. Caring for people, it's a way of life.

WRITING STYLES

There are many different styles of writing, ranging from romantic poetry to that used in a highly technical report. This section will provide an overview of the different types of writing style you are likely to need as a nurse. More detailed information on writing styles can be found in Fairbairn and Winch (1996), Powell (1999) and Rose (2001).

During your time as a student nurse, it is quite likely that you will be asked to use writing styles that are both technical and formal. For example, when writing patients' notes it is normal to use a formal style and there will be local guidelines that should be adhered to as well as the Nursing and Midwifery Council (NMC) professional guidelines for record keeping.

Look at the following entries in a patient's records.

- The patient looked like death. I tried to talk to her and ask her if she was OK but could not get out of her what the problem was, then the patient was sick all over the bed.
- The patient looked pale and unwell, and when asked if she was unwell she was unresponsive. The patient vomited a large amount of undigested food.

Notice how the second version is more formal and avoids using slang or colloquialisms. Spoken English is likely to contain colloquial words or phrases. Colloquial means ordinary or familiar as opposed to formal speech. Colloquial phrases make up 'everyday' English; however, such English also contains words that have a 'local' meaning. This form of English may be found only in a small or specific area of the UK; alternatively, it may be in general use in the UK but not in the English that is spoken in other parts of the world. For example, there are a number of words used to mean toilet, e.g. loo, WC, lav (short for lavatory), bog and rest room. Netty – a word used for toilet in the north east of England – is not used in any other part of the world. Understanding such phrases is important, as patients may use them; however, colloquial English should not be used when writing formal documents such as patients' notes or in academic work because its meaning may be misunderstood.

Writing in the third person

Formal writing is characterised by being rather impersonal because the author writes in what is called the *third person*. The more this style is used, the more impersonal the writing will seem. When writing in the third person the subject of the sentence (see p. 98) is not referred to directly. You will see this form of writing in its most extreme when you read scientific or medical research reports. If the third person is impersonal, what about the 'first' or 'second' person?

The 'first person' is used when you are referring to your own actions or those of a group to which you belong. When using the first person it is common to use the words *I* and *we*. In other words, you are describing the world from your point of view. The second person is a term used when the writer is talking to the reader. In this book we have used the second person when giving suggestions or recommendations; for instance, when we suggest that *you* should always arrive on time for lectures, we are using the second person.

The third person is where the subject (in grammatical terms) is not an identifiable individual and is often replaced with pronouns such as *it, he* and *they*. For example, when describing an experiment in the first person I would write: 'I put the water in the test tube.' However, when writing in the third person, this becomes: 'The water was put in the test tube.' Notice how in the second version the reader does not really know who put the water in the test tube, whereas in the first it is clear that it was me. Writing in the first person is commonly used when using reflection (see p. 185). When learning to write in the third person the trick is to remove any reference to individuals within the sentence. Words such as *I* or *we, they, he* or *she* should not be used; you need to be as impersonal as possible (Box 5.7).

Academic writing

Academic writing is a particular style of writing that is widely used in the academic and research world. It is an approach that is expected from individuals when they are presenting new ideas and thoughts that have been developed in an objective way. Academic writing style is used because it infers that the writer is being object-ive (considered all of the evidence without being biased) and has not influenced the outcome of research or investigation. The passive voice (third person or imper-sonal) is often used in relation to academic writing style. Academic style is formal and, as such, it avoids trying to be funny or light hearted. Sarcasm and irony are also not used, as the intention is to present knowledge and help others to under-stand, not to entertain (Box 5.8).

Box 5.7 Writing in the third person

Write a short paragraph about a recent event in your life, commenting on how you felt about the event.

Now re-write the paragraph in the third person without using the words 'I' or 'we' or referring to any 'proper nouns'.

Box 5.8 Academic writing style

This style of writing tends to have the following formal characteristics:

- Objective (unbiased)
- Analytical (breaks down issues into their component parts)
- Rational (based on the logical use of factual information)
- Balanced (doesn't give undue weight to a particular view)
- Logical
- Normally written in the third person but could be first person when reflecting on personal professional practice
- Avoids the use of colloquial English
- Uses standard English
- Systematic (tends to follow a predictable pattern of development)
- Scientific terminology
- Evidenced based (opinions and views are based on established facts)
- Referenced

When studying at university you will probably be encouraged to adopt an academic style, particularly for essays and research studies that you may be asked to do. When writing in academic style we use references or actual data to support what we are saying. Referencing is dealt with in Chapter 6 of this book.

As with most skills, you can improve you ability to write by observation, experience, practice and review. If you want to improve your ability to write in the third person, when you write you must ensure that there is no reference to you, the writer, in the sentences. So a sentence such as 'It would appear to me that schizophrenia is a treatable syndrome' becomes 'It would appear that schizophrenia is a treatable syndrome', and 'I asked the patient if he had any pain and he said no' translates to the third person as: 'When asked if he had any pain the patient said that he did not.'

When using an academic style remember that evidence is important, so you must constantly ask yourself questions such as: Who said that? Where did that thought come from? Where is the material to support that statement? It is also important to remember that academic writing should flow logically and any conclusions are based on an analysis and evaluation of the evidence (see Chapter 4). Lastly, if something really is just your opinion, say 'in my opinion'. If someone else has said it but you want to show that you agree, you can say, 'I support the view expressed by Ely and Scott (2006) that an academic style is more impersonal.'

Try to read two research-based articles each week; initially these could come from professional magazines such as the *Nursing Times* or *Nursing Standard*. Choose articles that are from the research sections rather than 'News' reports. As you read the articles, note the writing style and how and when it changes. See if you can spot where the author has an opinion but has used the third person.

When you are comfortable reading these articles, move on to articles from research journals. This type of activity will improve your own ability as a writer as well helping you discover new ideas about nursing practice. If you travel to college or your practice area by train or bus, these times can be used for this type of reading. Try practising converting first person to third person and third to first (harder).

Reflective style

Reflection is a way in which experiences are made sense of and learned from. Reflection is based on personal experience, and thus tends to be written in the first person.

> **Tip**
>
> When reflecting on your practice experience, remember to change the names of any patients and staff, and don't even mention the name of the ward or hospital. This is in accord with the NMC *Code of Professional Conduct* (NMC 2004).

If you are asked to reflect on your experience in an assignment, it is acceptable to write in the first person. The rules of academic style still apply, such as not using slang or informal terms, but when reflecting on professional practice it is acceptable to use the first person and this is seen in some books and journal articles. In general, when writing reflectively, descriptions of events and of emotions should be in the first person; analysis of the events and their evaluation should be written in the third person. If you are writing for an assignment, it is always a good idea to ask your tutor to confirm what their expectations are (see Chapter 8 for more on reflection).

Which tense to use

Deciding on which tense to use is sometimes difficult, particularly where a mix of reflective and academic styles is being used. This is even more difficult if you have been asked to develop action plans for your future development.

Reflective activities always tend to start with a description of an event that has happened, so clearly this type of writing should start in the past tense. This is also the case when describing activities in which you have taken part or witnessed. When writing about the work of others where conclusions have been made, again the past tense should be used. For instance, 'Johnson and Johnson (1909) found that massaging with certain oils made the skin feel much smoother.' Here you are reporting the findings of others; as these findings have been made in the past, past tense is appropriate. It is, however, common to use the present tense when introducing established ideas and concepts, such as 'Chicken pox *is* a common childhood illness.' The present tense can be used in this manner where there is no dispute about the fact of the information (for more detail, see Powell 1999). The present tense is normally also used when writing a set of instructions or giving a description of something.

Look at the small piece of reflection in Box 5.9. Notice how it starts in the past tense in the first paragraph where the description occurs but then moves into the present tense as the events are related to current research. Finally, the reflection ends with some suggestion for future action.

When writing reflectively, the past tense should be used for describing events and emotions, for analysing them and relating them to theory. However, as you move through the reflective cycle (see Chapter 8) you will start to consider what has been learned from your experience, and how this will affect your future practice and learning. In this final stage, you will start to use the future tense as you forecast what developments will occur.

What to avoid when writing

Communicating ideas and information is the prime reason for writing and thus being clear when you write is very important. When writing as a student or registered nurse, there are some features of language that are best avoided.

Jargon

Professional jargon means the terms and expressions that form the language used by a particular profession. Nurses may talk, for example, of a particular drug being given sub-cut; this is shorthand for a drug being given by injection subcutaneously. It is important to recognise the difference between jargon and that of

---

Box 5.9 Tenses and writing reflectively

Mr J had come to the clinic because he was suffering from hypertension. My mentor and I undertook a number of observations with Mr J (blood pressure, urinalysis, height and weight). My mentor advised Mr J that he was rather overweight (his body mass index was 29) and that this could be contributing to his hypertension. He was advised to start to take action to reduce his weight. My mentor checked with Mr J that he understood the types of food that he should eat less of, and that he did not want to see a dietian. When Mr J returned to the clinic 6 weeks later I was surprised to find that he had not lost any weight; in fact he had gain a kilo. I was rather disappointed in the patient and a little confused because I knew that he understood the problems and about eating a balanced diet. I discussed Mr J with my mentor who said that achieving their ideal weight was difficult for most patients because it meant changing their lifestyle.

With Mr J we had identified a problem and part of the solution, yet we had not properly supported Mr J to achieve the goals set for him. Research (Biggins 1999, Massoff 2001) suggests that weight loss will only be achieved and sustained when there is a change in lifestyle and that the patient's family, other networks and professionals must support this change. Thus for Mr J we must identify which aspects of his lifestyle we can help him change. Rogan and Josh (2002) contrast the support given (both formal and informal) to those who are trying to stop smoking and those who are trying to lose weight; they found that in all aspects the support available to dieters was lower in both terms of quality and quantity.

Following this incident, I have decided to investigate the factors that motivate people to lose weight and how those factors can be used to help people develop strategies for success.

All references are fictitious and are used for illustration purposes only.

---

specialised technical terms. Specialised technical terms are used to ensure precision and tend to be recognised by health professionals across the world. Jargon tends to evolve out of linguistic shortcuts and is likely to be recognised only relatively locally. In your professional life and your writing you will find that you will use jargon. It is important that you make sure that the person with whom you are communicating recognises and understands the jargon you are using. Similarly, when writing assessments, it is important that you explain the jargon you use, thus demonstrating that you understand what it means.

Use plain English

Writing in an academic style does not mean that you should write extended sentences using the longest words you can find! If possible, stick to short sentences and short words. If you do this the meaning of your sentences will be clear, and you will need to use much less punctuation. Look at the following sentence:

At this moment in time we are now in a position to refocus the remuneration scale, such that employees will observe a substantial elevation in their take home pay; this will be actuated from the first day of next month.

More simply:

From the 1st of next month, all staff will receive a big pay increase.

Notice how pompous the first sentence sounds: it uses phases where a single word would do, and has used longer words where a shorter one would do.

Words that have the same or similar meaning are called synonyms. They can be used to keep the language that we are using interesting. The English language has so many of these that special books called thesauruses have been created. A thesaurus indicates words with similar meanings. Although using synonyms can help to enliven your writing, if you use too many, your work will sound false. Not all synonyms are interchangeable and context is very important. In the first sentence, the word elevation has been used as a synonym of rise. But in a different sentence we could not use these words interchangeably (e.g. The house had an elevation of 6 metres).

Try to avoid the trap of being overcomplex and thus appearing pompous by always reviewing your work to see whether it can be expressed with greater simplicity. Given a choice of words to use, select the word that is used more commonly (normally the smaller word). Fairbairn and Winch (1996) provide some good and amusing examples of pompous and rather long-winded writing.

Stereotypes

It is a good idea to think about how we stereotype people from the outset of your career as a nurse. You will come across issues of diversity and equality wherever you work. When we write, we sometimes subconsciously use stereotypes. The most common example of this when discussing nursing is to write as if all nurses are female. For example: 'As in the past, the main responsibility of the modern nurse is to her patients.' This sentence assumes that all modern nurses are female, and could be rewritten as: 'As in the past, the main responsibility of modern nurses is to their patients.' It is worth asking the question when you read your work: Have I stereotyped anyone? In this way you will become more aware of issues surrounding equality and diversity.

> **Tip**
>
> The word 'their' is now often used instead of 'his' or 'her', although strictly speaking it should only be used in the plural, e.g. 'The men collected their coats.' Some people argue that it is better to use 'their' as using 'his' or 'her' in an attempt to avoid sexist language can become cumbersome. One way around this is to use plurals wherever possible, as we did in the sentence about modern nurses (see above).

GIVING PRESENTATIONS

Most courses will require you, at some point, to give an oral presentation. Some people seem to be naturally gifted at giving presentations – but don't despair, it is a skill that can be learned. While giving a presentation and giving a lecture are not exactly the same, it is worthwhile thinking about the various factors that make up a good lecture. A lecture should represent the art of oral presentation at its best. Remember, the purpose of a lecture is communication, not entertainment. In the context of education, an entertaining presentation is a good one only if you remember and understand the information it contained. Look at Box 5.10: do you recognise any of your lecturers?

Your tutors ask you to present your work because giving presentations forces you think about how information should be structured in order for it to be communicated. You can learn a great deal as you think about what to include and how to assemble a presentation. Preparing a presentation is part of the learning process; it is difficult to give a good presentation if you do not know what you are talking about. Therefore, in order to improve your presentation skills, you need to know and understand the subject you are presenting. If you really understand what you are talking about you will find that you are much less nervous.

Of course, the other important fact that your lecturers know only too well is that when you are doing a presentation you are exposed, so your classmates will know if you do not understand what you are delivering. Do not worry if you are concerned that your nerves will let you down, as your lecturers will be used to assessing nervous students.

Organisation

Next to understanding, being organised is probably the next most important thing. If your presentation is to be assessed, review the guidelines to that assessment, making sure you have covered all that you need to. Being organised has two sides: intellectual organisation and domestic organisation.

Box 5.10 Characteristics of a good lecturer

- Enthusiastic
- Well organised
- Knowledgeable
- Confident
- Admit when they do not know the answer
- Use clear visual aids
- Speak clearly

Intellectual organisation

To deliver a presentation you need to structure your ideas: you need an introduction, a middle section (development) and a conclusion (Fig. 5.2). This structure is like that of an essay, but when doing a presentation the combination of oral and non-verbal communication means that you can communicate in greater detail. You can also judge whether your audience is following what you are communicating.

The fact that your presentation needs a structure means that you must organise your thoughts and plan carefully what you want to say. Planning and structuring thoughts and arguments are discussed in other sections of this book, particularly with reference to note taking and essay writing (see Chapter 5). When thinking of structure you must consider such things as how much background information is required, important factual items to include, explanations, issues of contention, solutions to problems and other points of interest. Having a well-defined structure will also help you to keep to the point and remember the aim of your talk. Box 5.11 shows how a presentation about the measurement of blood pressure might be structured.

Introduction

An introduction must set the subject you are presenting in context; it also needs to inform the audience of why they should want to listen to you and what you hope they will achieve by listening (why you are talking to them). You need to outline what particular approach you will take. For example, in a presentation on the care of patients with pressure ulcers you may want to focus on current practice; alternatively, you may elect to base your talk on the latest research. Another approach would be to take a historical perspective, describing how and why practice has changed over the years. You may want to concentrate your talk about pressure ulcers in acute care settings rather than primary care settings; you may want to address the social care aspects of individuals rather than their direct health care needs. The introduction should be used to identify which particular aspects of the topic you will be addressing and the approach you will take.

It is also a good idea to let your audience know what the structure of the presentation will be. As you proceed with your talk you should always give clear indications to the audience as to where you are in a presentation. This 'signposting' helps those who have not been concentrating fully, and has also been shown to increase the amount of information that individuals retain (Brown & Atkins 1988).

Development

Your talk needs to develop in a logical manner; you need to establish the factual issues and support these with evidence. If you will be making inferences or

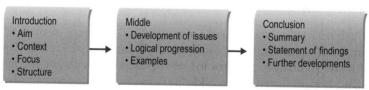

Figure 5.2 The structure of a presentation

Box 5.11 Example of a plan for a presentation

Introduction

Aim: To inform the audience of the practice of measuring blood pressure (BP), to raise some causes of error, to highlight future developments.

Context of talk: Largely acute settings, with recordings measured by practitioners.

Structure: Will follow the procedure and process. Will not look at any 'special circumstances'.

Specific points

1. Remind audience of origins of diastolic and systolic pressure and how it varies according to physiological state (based on O'Brien et al 1997). Use OHT of heart and circulation.
2. Client/practitioner interaction, introducing self, technique and obtaining consent (discuss role playing, obtaining consent).
3. Available equipment (slide of sphygmomanometer and common electronic devices with cuffs), go over equipment checks, discuss sizes. (Use example of cuff sizes in the US.)
4. Patient posture and position of arm/application of cuff, also position of equipment (slide of patient's arm, with cuff applied and stethoscope in position).
5. Nurse's posture/position, procedure and recording (flow diagram of process) – picture of chart.
6. Common sources of errors, posture, miss-cuffing, white coat hypertension (picture of me in white coat looking frightening).
7. Ambulatory blood pressure measurement – decline of the sphygmomanometer.

Conclusions

- Recording of BP is important and must be done with care
- Several potential causes of error
- Automated devices will replace sphygmomanometers, but...
- Ambulatory blood pressure measurement will become more important as technological improvement increasingly allows smaller, lighter devices to be designed

Use slide with bullet points and provide further reading.

---

deductions from the facts, these must be clearly linked to the facts that support them. Illustrate the points you are making with examples.

Most student presentations are about 10 minutes long. If you are going to use visual aids (and we recommend that you do) you need to think in terms of needing *no more* than seven overhead transparencies or slides. This limit includes those used for the title and gives you less than 2 minutes of presentation time per slide. Although it may appear that we have strayed into the realms of actually delivering the presentation, the point here is that the time you have available will dictate the number of points you can make or issues you can raise. If you also think in terms of one point per visual aid (e.g. overhead transparency), then the maximum number of points you can discuss in a 10-minute talk will be seven.

Once you have decided what to include you need to make sure that each point or issue discussed follows logically from the previous one. For example, if discussing the care of pressure ulcers it would seem sensible to discuss how the severity of the ulcer is assessed before discussing how it is treated and dressed.

Remember to include examples because examples illustrate the points you are making and help your talk to 'come alive'. Examples help your audience to relate to what you are saying and, if they can relate to your talk, they will enjoy it and are more likely to remember what you are saying. If discussing blood pressure measurement and cuff sizes you could use examples of where you had to use an extra large or very small cuff, or even bring them to show the audience.

Conclusion

Your conclusion should provide a summary of your main ideas. If your presentation was evaluative or contentious, it should include a statement of your principal findings, even if these may still be vague or tentative. For example, in Box 5.11 the conclusion was based on a summary and speculation of future developments. Finally, you can also indicate what further research or developments are needed or what developments are currently taking place.

Domestic organisation

Having organised and structured your thoughts ready for a presentation, the next thing you must do is organise the things you will need to support you, and work on your skills of delivery.

Rooms

If possible, familiarise yourself with the room where the presentation will take place. Stand at the front of the room to get an idea of what it will feel like when you are delivering the presentation, but also stand at the rear, so that you can appreciate what someone at the back of your audience will experience. If you will be using a projector it is worth doing this with the projector on. This will allow you to appreciate where you need to stand and again help you to appreciate what the audience will see. If you are going to use board pens (e.g. if you are going to work interactively with the audience), make sure that they work and that they are the correct type. White boards can be ruined if the incorrect pens are used on them. Check which colours are visible from the back of the room (red is notoriously difficult to read).

If you have time and you are able, consider arranging the seating in a way that will suit your approach. If you want to stimulate discussion, semi-circles are thought to work best, while having clusters of seats can stimulate group work. Fry et al (1999) provide useful information on seating arrangements and a variety of different approaches to presentations.

Visual aids

Visual aids mean things like overhead transparencies, PowerPoint presentations, flip charts, photographs and models or pieces of equipment. Visual aids should be used to help people learn. They sometimes take the form of notes; if you use bullet points, for example, you are telling the audience that you want them to note and remember the bullet points. On the other hand, visual aids are probably best deployed where they provide visual images of words, i.e. they are aimed at enhancing your verbal communications and are particularly useful for those whose dominant learning style is visual. Notice that, in the example of a presentation on blood pressure recording (see Box 5.11), most of the slides were images, not words. Avoid presenting pages of numbers, as the audience will gain little from them – use graphs or pie charts instead.

Explain each image you use to the audience. Your visual aids should enhance your talk and not just be there in the background. You must make the link between the visual aid and your verbal communications for the audience – they will not do it for themselves.

Do not put too much information onto each slide or overhead transparency. If you use text on your projections, use a font that is at least 24 pt. This also applies to any writing that you do on flipcharts. When using an overhead projector, place each transparency on the projector as if you are going to read it. Look at the projection screen and adjust the focus. Make sure the image is sufficiently large and that the projected image is square and not shaped like a tombstone (you may need to move the screen or the projector). You may need to clean the glass screen as well.

Think about where to stand so that you do not block out the image. If you want to refer to something specific on one of your transparencies you can point to it on the glass screen (Fig. 5.3). Overhead transparencies can be generated by computer,

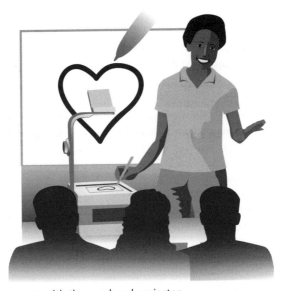

Figure 5.3 Using a pen with the overhead projector

by hand or by using a photocopier; your librarian or the staff based in media services will probably be able to help.

Computer programs

Computer software such as Microsoft's PowerPoint can be a great aid to putting a talk together. This software allows presentations to be assembled with ease. It has features such as animations, sounds, music and film clips that can be used to enhance presentations; it also links with other Microsoft software applications. The advantage of these packages is that not only do they make construction easier but they can also help liven up a presentation.

When using this and other presentation software, remember your audience. It is easy to get carried away producing a presentation that is technologically impressive, but difficult to follow because the substance of the talk is lost in the gimmicks of the presentation. For example, if you use different colours, remember that 10% of the male population is red–green colour blind. High contrast between the text on the slide and its background should be a goal; maximum contrast is achieved by using black on white.

Animations, while amusing, can become distracting, so use them sparingly and intelligently. Presentation software allows you to develop ideas by gradually revealing bullet points or arguments to discuss an issue, before revealing images that support it. Quite often the software will use a default size of text for headings and bullet points. It is a good idea to use the default settings because they are set at a size most people can read at a distance.

When using overhead slides or presentation software there are some simple rules:

- Use a large font size (minimum 24 pt) for text
- Keep your style consistent throughout
- High contrast (e.g. black on white) is great
- Keep it simple
- Explain each image as you use it
- Check out the technology before you use it
- Test your slides by standing at the back of the room to see if you can read them.

Speaking in public

Your aim is to convey the information and ideas that you have to the audience in a manner that will allow them to understand, retain and sometimes act on what you say. Think of it as an opportunity; when else do you get a chance to air your thoughts and views for 10 minutes or so without someone interrupting! When you give a presentation, you must speak clearly and slowly. It also helps if you are enthusiastic and display confidence because you know your subject.

Avoid reading directly from notes or the text of your talk, as this will force you to keep your head down. If you keep your head down your voice will not be projected and some of your audience will not hear what you are saying. A good technique that can help is to focus your eyes on something on the back wall of the room; this has the dual function of allowing your voice to be projected and removing the need to look at anyone in the audience. It is a good technique to use if you are nervous but can hinder the formation of a relationship with your audience. In addition, it does make it harder to look at any notes. Here a lectern can help; however, these are becoming relatively unusual. When you have gained confidence you will find it easier to make eye contact with your audience.

Tip

Making eye contact with your audience really helps to make them feel involved in your presentation. You should aim to 'look at someone all the time and everyone some of the time' when doing presentations.

Your voice needs to change tone as you speak. If you read from a prepared text this is less likely to happen and your talk may appear pedestrian and bland. You need to be loud enough to be heard, but not so loud that everyone would rather be in the next classroom! Try to avoid using local terms (colloquialisms) such as 'init' or 'you know what I mean' and do not use nursing slang or too many abbreviations; not everybody knows what COPD (chronic obstructive pulmonary disease) or NG tube (nasogastric tube) means.

Using notes

When giving a presentation most people will require some notes to prompt them as to what they are going to say next. Experienced speakers tend to use their visual aids as prompts, but when just starting you may want to use more structured notes. The most important thing to remember about notes is that you have to read them several times so you are familiar with them. If you try talking whilst looking at an audience and attempting to follow detailed notes at the same time you will soon see the problem.

One technique is to use notes with large, clear headings (14 pt) with clear bullet points to remind you of each issue. Using the example of the presentation about blood pressure (see Box 5.11) you may have:

Blood pressure
- Heart as pump. Pressure of blood in vessels = BP
- BP components – diastolic and systolic
  - Origins

This note reminds the speaker to talk about how blood pressure rises through the action of the heart pumping blood and that there are two recognisable stages (levels) of pressure associated with ventricular contraction and relaxation.

Using this technique you would have a note for each subsection of your presentation. If there are details that you feel you are likely to forget, highlight these in your notes and refer to them during your talk. The clear headings in the notes will help you to keep track of where you are in your talk.

Cue cards

An extension of this technique is to use cue cards. This is a technique whereby each note is placed onto a small card and, as the point is dealt with, the card is placed to one side. There is of course a danger that all the cards are dropped, so it is important to number each card. The advantage of cue cards it that, once a point is covered, the card can be put to one side, so it is easier to know where you are in your presentation.

Developing your technique

As discussed at the beginning of this section, there are two distinct aspects to doing a presentation. The first is about organising and structuring the presentation; the second concerns delivering the presentation itself. Organising and structuring information, debate and argument are skills that you will need for many types of communication and assessment. Improvement in these areas comes through practice, evaluation, self-reflection, peer review and observation. These techniques will also help with the delivery aspect. Through practice, you will develop a sense of how audiences respond, how they like to receive information and how this matches your style. Evaluation can come in several forms: it can be based on your own thoughts or those of others. Evaluation of your presentation should answer the following questions:

- What was good?
- What worked?
- Why did it work?
- What did not work? Why?
- What areas do I need to develop?

Sometimes it is difficult for us to evaluate our own performance because we are too emotionally involved with the event; it is in these circumstances that peer review can help. Peer review is based on the opinions of your peers, i.e. your fellow students. Your colleagues can provide good feedback and they will be able to have empathy with your situation. If you want to seek the views of your colleagues it is a good idea to ask them beforehand. This way they are aware that you are looking for a serious and considered view of your presentation, rather than just reassurance.

Video recording

Seeing yourself on video is a good way to examine your delivery skills; even though it feels scary, it is usually a really worthwhile experience. When watching a video of yourself, it is important to focus on aspects of your delivery and how to improve them (e.g. how you were positioned in relation to the projector), rather than how you looked. Audio recording can also be useful and may be easier to arrange.

SUMMARY OF KEY POINTS

- Being able to write well is important in your clinical placements as well as in your academic work.
- Spelling accurately is important. Computer spell checkers and grammar checkers can be really helpful but it is important to check the meaning of words.
- Careful attention to punctuation is important as it can change the meaning of a sentence.
- The apostrophe is often misused – only use it in place of missing letters or when indicating ownership.
- The English language is dynamic and conventions (e.g. the use of capital letters) change over time.
- Reflective writing skills are important in nursing and many of your assessments will require this. Use of the first person is expected in reflective writing but is less common in academic writing.
- Oral presentations require the same structure as an essay. Preparation of the room and equipment in advance of the presentation can help you relax.
- Oral presentations really demonstrate your understanding (or lack of it!) of a topic.
- Although daunting, video recording can provide excellent feedback on your technique, style, etc.

6

How to pass assessments

Learning objectives

This chapter will help you learn how to:

- Write good essays with appropriate and accurate references
- Prepare effectively for written exams
- Develop good techniques for a viva or practical exam
- Prepare a poster
- Pass your practice-based assessments
- Make effective use of feedback from markers.

INTRODUCTION

Your programme will contain a number of assessments (sometimes referred to as coursework or assignments) in one form or other. The main purpose of assessments is to determine whether learning has taken place and that you have acquired the knowledge, skills and attitudes needed to register as a nurse. These are necessary not only to meet the competencies that are required of a registered nurse, set in the UK by the Nursing and Midwifery Council (NMC), but you must also be shown to be of 'good character and in good health'. Therefore you must have demonstrated a professional attitude in your behaviour during your time as a student and be fit to practise. In the UK those responsible for your programme are required to sign a statement to testify that you have achieved the course outcomes and that you are of good character and in good health before you can register with the NMC. For further information, visit the NMC website at www.nmc-uk.org.

Assessments and tests are a necessary part of your learning and have to be passed to complete the course successfully. Your course is likely to include some written examinations, projects and extended essays, which are designed to test a wide range of knowledge and understanding as well as your organisational skills and your ability to write records of patient care. You will probably also be required to undergo practical examinations whereby your performance is tested. These may occur in the skills laboratory, in class when you give a seminar presentation and in practice when your practical skills with real patients can be observed. This chapter is designed to help you manage your assessments effectively in order that you can do well. Preparation for oral presentations such as lectures and seminars is covered in Chapter 5.

PREPARING FOR ASSESSMENTS

There are several ways to improve your chances of passing assessments. One of the most valuable assets you can acquire is a positive attitude, so do not see assessments as traps to make you fail but as an opportunity to achieve. Essays and exams (assessments) are features of university courses but unfortunately many adults have negative thoughts about these, particularly exams – often a legacy from their school years. These attitudes should be firmly put aside.

Studying the subject is clearly essential, but by developing appropriate writing techniques for the different types of exams and essays you encounter in your programme, you will be more likely to gain a good grade. Be proactive and find out exactly how you will be tested as this will help reduce anxiety about assessments. Exams can be especially stressful; however, the root of anxiety about exams is fear of failure, and this needs to be recognised and then effectively managed with good preparation. Fear can be very destructive and can result in us becoming convinced that we will fail (Hadley 1999). In addition, fear can make us become irrational; remember, you would not have been accepted to undertake your nursing programme if you did not have the potential to succeed.

The essential first step for all assessments is making sure you understand what is required. Start from the point when you are given the assessment information so that you do not waste time. At this early stage, make sure you look at the marking criteria; this will be in your handbook or with the assessment information. Some parts of the required answer may be considered more important and therefore allocated more marks. Knowing how the marks will be allocated will guide you to include relevant material of the required quantity and help you avoid including material that will only attract a small percentage of the mark. Discuss the required content with your personal tutor.

Writing essays

The essay is a common form of assessment on university courses. It requires students to present a reasoned argument, supported by references to relevant theory. Essays are short or long prose discussions which are used by authors to consider arguments on a subject. In general literature they are used to inform, amuse and discuss issues, often including the personal viewpoints of the writer. However, when writing an essay at university as part of your course work, different things are required. You will be expected to write in a formal academic style with the intention of critically analysing issues as a test of your knowledge and understanding: you are not expected to entertain the person marking your essay.

> **Tip**
>
> Never try to be funny when writing an academic essay – tutors will not be amused!

Essay structure

Essays should be structured with an introduction to tell your readers what to expect in the essay, the main body, which should contain your arguments, and a conclusion to end the essay by identifying the main issues. An essay will test your knowledge of the issues taught during a unit of learning, module, term or part of the programme. Students often wonder how essay writing is relevant to bedside nursing. As well as testing what you have learned, the skill of writing is also important because maintaining records is an essential part of nursing and increasingly nurses are required to produce comprehensive reports that could possibly be used in a court of law. Nurses need to be able to justify their actions and demonstrate that they are able to link their practice to current research.

Getting started – essay timetables

Not knowing where to start often deters students from working on their essays. It may seem difficult to know where to start, so do this by planning a timetable for completing the essay. Create your timetable (Table 6.1) as soon as you are given your assessment guidelines. Plan to start work immediately and aim to finish at

Table 6.1 Essay timetable

When	What to do	How long
Start 12 weeks from final submission date	Read essay guidelines Note exactly when and where the essay has to be handed in (make a note in your diary or planner)	This will probably take about an hour depending on the length of your assessment guidelines
Week 1	Clarify the task; discuss this in your study group and with your personal tutor Check you understand the focus of the essay and the weighting of each point Arrange a time when your tutor can read your first draft	2–3 hours
Weeks 2–3	Search for information, definitions and key texts Allow time for library books to become available if they have to be reserved, although there may be a reference copy in the library	5–15 hours
Week 4	Plan an outline of the structure of the essay by brainstorming headings for the main sections You can then break these up with subheadings for smaller subsections	This may take some time so allow 3–5 hours
Weeks 5–6	Write sections/subsections (create your reference list as you go) to produce your first draft	It is best to do one section at a time, aiming to write about 200–400 words in 1–2 hours
Week 7	Check your assignment guidelines again to make sure you have addressed the task Plan to leave your work for a few days then edit the main body – check references as you edit	1–2 hours
Week 8	Ask for tutor's comments	It may take about 1–2 weeks to get comments back
Week 9	Write second draft and check references Again leave your work for a few days before going on to the next stage	2–3 hours
Weeks 10–11	Edit second draft and write final version of the essay	2–3 hours
End of Week 11	Be ready to hand in with all the required documents	
Week 12	Hand in on time!	

least a week before the final submission date. When you create this timetable it is essential that you allow enough time for attention to detail so that you do not end up working to unrealistic deadlines.

> **Tip**
>
> A guide to calculating how long written work will take is to guess how long it will take to write up, edit and proofread your work, then double it as it is likely to take at least twice as long as you originally estimated!

After you have written one essay you will have a clearer idea but for your first essay be guided by the stages outlined below and discuss these with your personal tutor. The length of an essay will dictate how long it will take you to plan, research, write and then finally edit your essay: an approximate guide for a 2000 word essay with a 12-week period to reach completion might be between 20 and 30 hours for all of the activities associated with producing the finished essay.

You can see from Table 6.1 that essay writing needs time and you still have to be aware that you may be at the mercy of mechanical breakdowns such as printer failure and corrupted computer discs. These problems do happen and seem to be more likely to occur when you are pressed for time! You may have more than one assessment to work on at any one time such as exams or other assignment tasks. This will require careful planning to ensure you are working on the aspects that are a priority and meeting all deadlines. If you have to work on more than one assessment, keep a careful record of submission dates in your diary.

If you are not used to writing long essays, just the thought of writing 2000 words or more can be overwhelming; even experienced students find the idea of a long essay a challenge. The answer is to plan each step and break down your main task into smaller manageable tasks which are not so scary. To be asked to write an essay of 2000 words may seem a large task but tackling ten smaller sections of 200 words at a time can make it more manageable.

> **Tip**
>
> The process of essay writing will include finding information, drafting and revision: do not expect to just write the material from start to finish without revisions. Write up your reference list as you go (see pp. 139, 147); this activity can sometimes take almost as much time as writing the essay and leaving it to last will put you under additional pressure.

Planning your essay

Structure and direction are essential when writing an essay. This means your essay management strategy should start by focusing on planning. A good plan will help to create a sound framework and this structure will be obvious to the reader. A step-by-step approach is needed. The following steps may sound laborious but will help to ensure that the finished essay is comprehensive and free from errors.

Keeping focused on the essay title or task

It is important to keep focused on the essay title or assignment task to avoid getting sidetracked and not providing the material that the markers are looking for in your essay. Your assignment task may be in the form of a question such as 'Discuss the strategies a nurse may utilise to overcome difficulties when communicating with patients in a clinical environment'. Here the focus of the essay is clear, i.e. you need to consider a range of strategies that can be used to communicate effectively with patients in a clinical environment.

Alternatively, you may be given a more general task such as 'Reflect upon your placement experience'. Although this is not phrased as a specific question you still need to ensure that each section of the essay is focused on this task. Check the marking guide if there is one, as this will give more detail of what is required and make sure you attend any sessions related to the task. If you are not sure about what is required, seek clarification from your tutors. Assignments normally test the student on the learning that should have occurred during part of or the whole of the course. The essay is therefore a test of what you have learned.

- Check your handbook to find out the aims of the course, module or unit of learning. Aims are a general statement of intent and these will indicate the broad area of what you should have learned.
- Then look at the learning outcomes or objectives (statements of what you are supposed to have learned by the end of the course or unit of learning).
- Next consider the content, i.e. what you have been taught (look back at your timetables and notes).
- Finally, look at the essay guidelines and make the connections between what you should have learned and what you are supposed to write in your essay. Check the weighting (how the marks are allocated) for each aspect of the essay.

By the end of this thinking phase you should be able to identify the most important issues to include in the essay. In educational terms, to achieve a pass you must demonstrate that you understand the key issues and can apply principles to ensure safe practice.

Check your lecture notes

The points to include in the essay should have been covered in your lectures, therefore check your notes and handouts. If you have missed any lectures then you may have missed key issues and recommended reading. Check with friends or see the lecturer concerned or access their website.

There are usually specifically recommended texts and other materials for each module or unit of learning and this is where you might start the next phase – planning the essay – which involves looking for information.

Use keywords and definitions as a starting point

Once you have identified key areas of content you need to search for information. Use all available learning resources (see Chapters 2 & 3). Your thinking should have identified keywords to explore by looking for definitions of these terms. Nursing dictionaries, rather than general English dictionaries, should be used as they provide clear definitions of nursing-related terms, which can form the basis of further discussion. Use the larger versions of nursing dictionaries in the library, rather than pocket dictionaries, to give you a wider range of ideas. Other specialist dictionaries such as a dictionary of sociology or a dictionary of research may prove helpful.

Definitions can help clarify your thoughts and give you more keywords with which to search (see p. 61). Even at this early stage you need to start making careful notes of the sources of your references. Good referencing (see pp. 112, 139) comes from keeping full and systematic records of all publication details; you do not want to waste time searching for publication details at a later date.

> ### Tip
> Whenever you are reading books and journals or websites, always make a note of the full reference details at the time; it will save hours of searching later if you decide to use the material in your essay. Keep the information about your references on reference cards or on a computer.

Plan your arguments

In everyday speech an argument has often come to mean 'a fight'; however, in academic terms, arguments are a series of reasoned ideas that support a point of view. The strength of an argument will help you form judgements. As a registered nurse practitioner you will have to make decisions about the type of care a patient will receive and you must learn to select appropriate actions. A critical discussion should be incorporated in your plan for your essay rather than simply regurgitating information without considering whether there are any alternative points of view.

Create an overall plan of the essay

The next stage is putting things together for your overall plan to get the structure of your essay clear. Imagine that the structure of the essay is like a framework that supports the material you are presenting. Using notes from lectures and your own searches in the library, start putting ideas in the form of headings or bullet points into a sequence. To achieve this you can either work with a large sheet of paper with self-adhesive notes or small slips of paper or use the computer. Move the ideas around into what looks like a logical order and then create your written plan of the main sections of the essay; these can then be subdivided into smaller subsections of the essay (Box 6.1). Do not worry about writing the introduction or conclusion: just have them as headings as it is more important at this stage to ensure your essay has a clear structure.

Box 6.1 Essay plan

Essay main body – Communication

- Verbal communication (section)
  - Oral communication
  - Written communication
- Non-verbal communication (section)
  - Signs and symbols
  - Eye contact
  - Gestures
  - Touch
  - Body posture
  - Proximity

Plan subsections

When you have a rough idea of the subsections you can plan each one in more detail, noting keywords or concepts that should be included. Make sure that the material follows a logical order and that there are links between the last sentence of one paragraph and the first of the next. Avoid short paragraphs that are merely statements but do not explain issues.

Planning the introduction

Do not worry about your introduction at this stage; write two or three sentences simply stating what the essay will be about and leave it until you have finished the first draft of the main body. Students often struggle to write an introduction as the first thing they do when writing the essay. Consequently, they spend far too long on a section of the assignment that may not receive many marks in proportion to the effort expended upon it. Introductions can be left until last because by then you know exactly what you have included in your essay.

Main body of the essay

The whole essay needs to be kept in mind while working on each section. Remember the main question posed by the essay to prevent you going in the wrong direction. This can happen when you find a large amount of information relating to a subsection which is in too much detail. Your essay plan will help you keep the whole essay in mind while you work on the subsections. However, do not worry if you have too much material in the first draft stage as this can be edited out later.

Keeping within the word limit

You will need to learn the academic skill of being concise in your written work as this is why word limits are imposed. The assignment instructions normally set a word limit which often allows a 10% margin, e.g. for a 2000 word essay you should not write more than 2200 words. You will be penalised (by only being awarded a borderline pass regardless of the quality of your work) if you exceed the word limit and in some universities markers will refuse to mark your work. If you write a lot less than the word limit you may not be penalised but you are unlikely to achieve a pass grade.

Assessment regulations are there to ensure that everyone is treated in the same way, i.e. it's fair to everyone and no students are allowed to benefit from unequal treatment. If you were allowed to go over the word limit you would have an unfair advantage over your fellow students who had kept to the word limit. Always check exactly what material is excluded from the word limit: the list of references at the end of the essay is not normally counted. When writing your essay using the computer it is easy to check your word total using the Tools menu. Get to know what 100 typed and handwritten words look like so you have an approximate idea of how much you have written. Check your guidelines for the main focus of the essay and allow more words for that than other sections.

Appendices

An appendix (plural appendices) is an additional item that appears after the text. Only include items in an appendix if you are instructed to do so in the guidelines. Do not try to use an appendix to circumvent the word limit regulations. If it is relevant it should be in the essay. Extra material in an appendix cannot be given marks, as this would mean that words, if added to your essay, would exceed the word limit. If, however, the guidelines stipulate that you should include charts or articles as an appendix, put these after the references. If you have more than one appendix, number them in sequence.

Hand written versus word-processed drafts

When drafting an essay by hand always start a new sheet of paper for each section and only write on one side of the paper. This will enable you to cut up the pages to rearrange passages of your work at a later date. You may soon realise that writing by hand is more time consuming and should aim to move to writing your essays on the computer as soon as possible.

If you are using a computer, insert page breaks between the sections. This will allow you to work on more than one section at a time: you do not have to work sequentially and if you find one bit difficult, try working on another. Headings could be regarded as a matter of taste. Some academics do prefer them as they signpost the essay, whereas others simply do not like them and prefer text without headings. If you find headings useful, you can work with them in the text but omit them when you get to the final version.

Using direct quotes

A direct quote means copying the exact words from a book or article and quotation marks ('') must be used to indicate that it is a direct quote. As a general rule you should use direct quotes with care. They are a bit like salt in a dish of food; a little is important for flavour but too much will ruin the taste. A quote needs to be used for a purpose and this should be clear to the reader; do not include a quote in the text without explaining why it is there. A short quote of a few words may illustrate an idea but longer quotes should be discussed to show the relevance of the material to your essay.

Never put one quote after another with no discussion. Such a strategy tends to give the marker the impression that you are a bit short of ideas and does not demonstrate an understanding of the issues involved. You may have been used to including a lot of quotes when studying subjects such as English Literature when discussing a play or poem, but with nursing it is important to paraphrase (put into your own words) to demonstrate understanding and use quotes in moderation.

Students often ask, 'How many quotes should you use in an essay?' This depends on the length of the essay but a good rule is when you use direct quotes use them sparingly – no more than two (or at the most three) direct quotes per 1000 words. Keep direct quotes short, never more than two or three sentences. The problem with too many long direct quotes is that they use up the word limit without gaining a corresponding number of marks.

Presenting quotes in your text

Quoted material can be run into the sentence, for example: It is important to keep blood in "…a special refrigerator at 2–6 degrees C to prevent contaminants reproducing" (Nicol et al 2004: 88). This is best done when only a few words are used.

Complete sentences should be distinguished by using italics and preferably indentation of the text to make it clear that it is a quote:

Adult education is a collaborative, transactional encounter in which objectives, methods and evaluation should be negotiated by all concerned.

(Brookfield 1986: 126)

Or by using quotation marks as follows:

"Adult education is a collaborative, transactional encounter in which objectives, methods, and evaluation should be negotiated by all concerned"

(Brookfield 1986, p. 126)

As you will see in the examples above, when you use a direct quote it is essential that you include the page number after the date indicated either by a 'p' or a colon (:).

Having warned you to be careful with quotes, there are circumstances when it is appropriate to use direct quotes. You should use direct quotes if the author has said it so succinctly that it is difficult to paraphrase. For example, Florence Nightingale's words concerning hospitals "should do the sick no harm" (Nightingale 1863, cited by Baly 1991) are often used. Famous quotes do show an awareness of nursing literature and are a good way of adding a touch of style to an academic essay.

Definitions should always be direct quotes and these are good for providing a starting point when discussing an essay. For example, if you were writing an essay about nursing models you might like to begin the body of your essay with a quote such as:

A nursing model is made up of the components or ideas that go towards making up nursing – what it is, its beliefs and values, and the theories and concepts on which it is built.

(Pearson et al 2005: 29)

The alternative to quoting verbatim is to paraphrase what the author (or authors) has said. Although a few quotes are good, more marks are likely to be given if you have paraphrased the idea and referred to two or more authors who agree or disagree with the issue under discussion.

Referencing – getting it right

Good referencing is a must. You cannot write academically unless you have mastered the skill of referencing. Therefore referencing is an important skill you need to acquire. The basis for good essays is accurate referencing. If you do not acquire this skill you will never get good marks. Poor or inaccurate referencing is nearly always a contributing factor in a failed essay. If you publish material which is incorrect it may cause difficulties when your reader searches for information electronically (Oermann & Ziolkowski 2002). Correct referencing can dramatically increase your chances of gaining a pass grade.

Find out which system is required by your university. It is likely that you will be given a guide or told to use a specific format; make sure you have these guidelines to hand when writing references. Although it may seem a bit difficult at first, with practice it will become, like many nursing procedures, much easier. Most references are straightforward but occasionally you may find something that is not clear, such as some surnames which are hyphenated or articles in journals which have no author. When you are compiling your references and you encounter an item that you are not sure how to reference, check with your reference guide, personal tutor or librarian.

What is a reference or citation?

You demonstrate your knowledge in an essay by using ideas from published material which are explicitly referred to in your text. This can either be by quoting directly from the source, i.e. using the exact words an author (or authors) has used, or paraphrasing, i.e. summarising in your own words what an author (or authors) has said. The process of referencing has two parts:

- A reference or citation, which is an indication of the source of the ideas in the text
- The list of source details at the end of the essay.

Therefore, in the context of an essay, a 'reference' means acknowledging the authors whose work you have used when developing your arguments in your essay. All references should be listed at the end of the essay. Referencing may be called citing and a reference may also be referred to as a 'citation'.

A reference list needs to provide the full publication details of each reference. These are not included in the text as this would be distracting for the reader but the reader must have these details to enable them to check the sources for themselves. The key details are indicated in the text by either a number (Vancouver style) or by giving the author's surname and year of publication and, if a direct quote, the page number (Harvard style).

The reference list at the end of your text should be presented using a recognised referencing system. A referencing system is a set format of writing the publication details of the books, journals or websites. There are a number of different referencing systems, some of which are more usually used in specific subjects. The most commonly used are the Harvard and the Vancouver systems.

> **Tip**
>
> You will improve your understanding of referencing by examining how this is done in the books and journals that you read. Make a point of noting how referencing is done in printed works.

The Harvard system

The Harvard system is more often used in academic work. This system uses the author's surname (without initials) and the date of publication in the text of the essay. These surnames, followed by the author's initials, are given with full publication details in alphabetical order in a reference list at the end of the essay. In the Harvard system references are not numbered either in the text or in the reference list (see Box 6.3).

You may find that there are some slight variations of the Harvard system. Therefore you *must* follow precisely the conventions of the Harvard system required by your university and not create a hybrid form of referencing. If you fail to reference correctly you will lose marks as your reader will not be able to verify that you have correctly cited an author's work. There are some variations in the Harvard system that you may see when reading reference lists in books and journals, as publishers often have their own choice of style. Generally, you should check your course handbook to see what style is required and follow the guidelines for this rigidly.

The Vancouver system

The Vancouver system is often used in what is known as 'quick read journals' where the flow of the reader's attention is less likely to be interrupted. It uses superscript numbers in the text to denote a reference and these are listed in numerical order at the end of the text. This system is generally not recommended for academic essays. Discuss this with your tutor if you are unsure which system is acceptable.

> **Tip**
>
> Until you get used to referencing, keep your guide with you when note taking or writing an essay so that you get into the habit of doing it correctly.

Although students often regard referencing as an end task to tidy things up, referencing is a more fundamental process. Organising your references should start as soon as you start reading. It is a practice that should become second nature, just the same as hand washing. Whenever you read something and take notes, then take a full reference at the same time.

In our experience students that reference well are those that have grasped the fundamental importance of knowledge to learning. They have not only grasped the importance of that knowledge but have also started to understand how our knowledge and understanding of the modern world comes about.

The importance of understanding the 'sources of knowledge' to studying is why we have given prominence to referencing. By using a wide range of reading material you will be able gain an in-depth knowledge of nursing; however, as you read you must keep references. When you write assignments you will use these references to help demonstrate your knowledge.

When citing an author (or authors), you are introducing theoretical ideas into your essay and this is how you demonstrate your knowledge. If your text has no explicit theoretical ideas that are attributable to a source, your reader is bound to question the validity of your information. For example, if you describe a nursing procedure but fail to refer to or cite an author (or authors) who advocates this practice, your reader may well question whether the method is supported by recent research. Alternatively, and what is more likely, they will think you have copied work direct from a text, which is an example of plagiarism (see p. 216). Therefore, you need to show that you know not only what you are doing but also *why* you are doing it by referring to theory.

To stress this vital point again, you should start writing references *before* you start writing your assignments, i.e. record all of the sources you have used and keep them in a file in 'reference format' when you acquire the information. This means that when you take notes from written sources you always take the full reference to go with those notes, thus ensuring that you have all the publication details required for your reference list.

For books, note the page numbers of the passages of interest. It is also useful to note the library where you found the book, as well as the catalogue number. Although this information is not needed for the reference list, it will save time if you need to locate the book again. Even if it is not what you are looking for at that particular time, it might be useful at a future date. You will never remember later where an article or book was even if you think you will at the time. Preferably, you should keep all your references electronically so that when you find you need a reference again, e.g. in a subsequent assignment, all you have to do is transfer the reference from one file to another.

If you do not have a computer an alternative method is to use an indexed book or index cards (Fig. 6.1). The first part of this card is the reference as it would appear in the list, the second is for your own information. The card can either be used to provide a direct quote, which it is why noting page numbers is important, or alternatively you might decide to paraphrase the idea.

How does referencing affect the grade given to an essay?

Marks are gained when work is correctly referenced; however, marks are lost when there are errors in referencing such as missing references, which means that surnames are cited in the text but not included in the reference list. Citing an author's name but not giving the reference is a serious error. You must allow time in your assignment schedule to check text references against your reference list.

Communication – anxiety in care environments
Sully, P. and Dallas, J. (2005) Essential Communication
Skills for Nurses
Edinburgh: Elsevier Mosby.

(University Main Library – number WP 243)
"Most people admitted to a care environment are likely
to experience a degree of anxiety" p36

Figure 6.1 Example of a reference card

If your work lacks specific references to the theory you are discussing it will not gain marks. If you have copied ideas or exact text but not referenced these ideas you will not only lose marks but you will be plagiarising, i.e. stealing ideas and presenting them as your own. A potentially good essay can be badly let down by inaccurate referencing; on the other hand, a well-referenced essay will create a positive impression and can gain valuable marks.

How many references does an essay need?

A question often asked by students is, 'How many references do I need to include in an essay?' Although this may seem like reducing an essay to a formula, students who are novices at writing long essays often value a guideline until they have become more experienced at constructing arguments. Therefore do not worry if at first you feel you need some idea of how many references to include. There is a simple answer to this question: if a statement you have made needs a reference it *must* go in. Setting a specified number of references should not detract from the importance of understanding the material. However, a general rule that may help you when you start writing essays at degree or diploma level is that you should have about eight to ten references for every thousand words. This might sound a lot but it is only one reference per hundred words.

An assignment of 2000 words that has fewer than five references is highly unlikely to achieve a pass grade, as there would be insufficient supporting material from published ideas. It would also indicate to the marker that you have not 'read around' your subject. If you feel unsure about this, ask your personal tutor for advice.

Types of references

The range of material used is also important. You should have in your reference list a range of literature in which there are both established ideas (generally found in textbooks) and more current research (generally found in recently published journals). However, some journal articles are considered seminal works (those that are the source of original ideas) and may be over 20 years old; in addition, textbooks are now updated more regularly. You may need to use a range of general nursing journals or specialist journals.

Recent material is important in clinical issues as many clinical practices become quickly outdated by new innovations or research. Clinical issues should normally have been published within the last 3–5 years. Therefore, when using theory, you must consider when it was published and whether it is still current. Alternatively, there may not have been anything published on an issue in 10 years. If you are not sure how current a clinical issue is, check with your subject tutors or placement staff. On the other hand, a theory may be still relevant even if it has not been recently published; for example, when citing psychological theory you may refer to work published in the first half of the twentieth century.

Introducing references

Your essay can be tedious to read if you simply state that this author 'said' this and that author 'said' that. You need to use a variety of phrases in your essay to give more vitality to your work. Box 6.2 shows some examples of other ways to introduce references in your work.

Box 6.2 Examples of phrases for introducing references

Andrews and Patterson (1999) introduced the concept of …
As stated by Pak (2000) …
Somas (2001) indicates that …
A perspective considered by Miles (2002) is one which …
Charleston and Dance (2005) suggest that …
Apio (1998) identified …
Alternatively, Rucker (2002) shows …
Kohen (2004) demonstrates …
Singh and Johnson (2001) outlined …
Stoker and Michael (2004) argue that …
(NB: All names are fictitious and used for illustration purposes only.)

Using an indirect reference

This is where the reference is included at the end of the sentence to indicate the source of the material that you have used. The author's name followed by the publication date are all given inside the brackets. The closing bracket is then followed by a full stop as shown in this example (NB: the reference is for illustration purposes only): Eye contact is important when conversing with patients; however, in some cultures eye contact may not always be appropriate in conversations between people of different family or social status (Janas 2000).

General rules for references in the text

Surnames only are used, not initials or first names. If the names are unfamiliar to you, check with the librarian. If there is a hyphen then both surnames are stated, e.g. Brastead-Jones (2000). If there is no hyphen only the last name is used. Dates are given by year; if the same author has published two different items in the same year you denote these by a lower case letter, e.g. Janas (2000a), Janas (2000b), and this also appears in the reference list.

If there is no named author, the organisation or journal becomes the author; for example, an unnamed article in the Nursing Standard would be written as Nursing Standard (2000). Organisations can be both authors and publishers, e.g. Nursing and Midwifery Council (NB: Names are fictitious).

Referencing an edited book

If you are new to the idea of referencing this is where it might get a bit complex. An edited book means that a variety of authors may have written the chapters but this has all been reviewed and drawn together by the editor(s). The editor(s) may also have written some of the chapters or none at all. The chapter authors' names

---

Box 6.3 Example of a reference list

BBC-BBCi-Homepage. *The home of the BBC on the internet.* http://www. bbc.co.uk. (Accessed 9 April 2003).

Brooker, C. and Nicol, M. eds. (2003) *Nursing adults: the practice of caring.* Edinburgh: Mosby.

Clarke, C. (2000) Children visiting family and friends on adult intensive care units: the nurses' perspective. *Journal of Advanced Nursing,* 31(2): 330–338.

Dale, A. E. (2005) Evidence-based practice: compatibility with nursing. *Nursing Standard,* 19(40): 48–53.

Druskat, V. and Wolff, S. (2001) Building the emotional intelligence of groups. *Harvard Business Review,* 79(3): 80 [Online] Business Source Premier. Available at http://www.ebsco.com/home. (Accessed 25 April 2003).

Fairbairn, G. J. and Fairbairn, S. A. (2001) *Reading at university.* Buckingham: Open University Press.

Greenhalgh, T. (2001) *How to read a paper – the basics of evidence-based medicine.* 2nd ed. London: BMJ Publications.

Heseltine, K. and Edlington, F. (1998) A surgery post-operative telephone call line. *Nursing Standard Online,* [online] 10(9). http://nursing-standard. co.uk/vol13-09/research.htm. (Accessed 23 November 1998).

Hull, C., Redfern, L. and Shuttleworth, A. (2005) *Profiles and portfolios – a guide for health and social care.* 2nd ed. Basingstoke: Palgrave Macmillan.

Nursing and Midwifery Council (2004) *The NMC code of professional conduct: standards for conduct, performance and ethics.* London: NMC.

Thayre, K. and Peate, I. (2003) Coping with expected and unexpected death. In: Hinchcliff, S., Norman, S. and Schober, J. eds. *Nursing practice and health care.* 4th ed. London: Arnold.

White, A. R., Rampes, M. and Ernst, E. (1999) *Acupuncture for smoking cessation* (Cochrane review) [CD ROM] The Cochrane Library. Issue 4. Oxford: Update Software.

Winston, R. (1998) *The human body: Part 1, Life story.* 50 min. [Videocassette]. London: BBC.

will appear in the contents list and (sometimes) at the beginning of the chapter, but not on the front of the book. However, the ideas will be the intellectual property of the chapter author so when you write your reference in the text you must state the chapter author, not the editor. Box 6.3 shows how an edited book is stated in the reference list.

Using primary and secondary sources

A primary source is the publication where a new piece of information or idea is first recorded. These primary sources are often used in other publications, when they are referred to as secondary sources. If you read a book by Janas, who in the text refers to an idea by Peterson, you have two options. In the book by Janas you will find the reference for Peterson and you can use this to check the original idea in Peterson's work. Realistically, however, if you are doing an assignment, you might not have time to find the book or article by Peterson or it may be out of print or difficult to obtain. In this case you can still use Peterson's idea (the primary source) but make it clear you found this idea in the book by Janas (secondary source). Therefore, in the text of your essay you would say: 'Janas (2000) citing Peterson (1968)' or 'Peterson (1968) as cited by Janas (2000)'. Although it is acceptable to use secondary sources, be careful about doing this repeatedly in your essay. If the primary source is easily available in the library your marker will not be impressed. In the reference list only the book you have used (the secondary source) would be listed (NB: Names are ficitious).

The reference list and bibliography

The reference list should contain the publication details of all the materials you have referred to in your text. A bibliography is a name sometimes used for a reference list; however, a bibliography can also be a term used to show general reading related to the subject but not actually referred to in the text. It is best to check your university guidelines as to what they want included in a bibliography, if this is required at all.

> **Tip**
>
> Do not embellish your reference list with different styles of brackets – keep it plain.

The Harvard system requires the author's surname followed by initials and then the date in brackets. This is followed by the title of the book. If it is a journal article the title of this is given followed by the journal title. Titles of books or journal titles are highlighted by using either italics or underlining; the title of the article is not highlighted. For books, if it is a second or subsequent edition, the edition is noted after the title; first editions are not noted. The place of publication of the book (town or city) is followed by the name of the publisher. The publisher's name is usually followed by the place of publication on the title page of the book. If there is more than one place of publication indicated on the title page, the first place name is normally taken as the place of publication.

Managing a reference list on a computer

When you start writing your essay it is a good idea to create a separate file for your reference list. Normally a reference list is not counted towards the essay word count. However, you should check this with your tutor/university assessment regulations. Having a separate document for the essay will allow you to check the number of words you have written accurately to ensure you do not exceed the word limit. As you insert references in the text of your essay, go to the second file and write the full reference in your reference list. This will save time later as writing out a reference list can take longer than most students allow. It also reduces the likelihood of missing references, which may cause you to lose a significant amount of marks.

> ### Tip
>
> When using a separate file for references for your essay, use single spacing and leave a line between each reference. When all are listed, save the document and then use the 'sort' command (e.g. the Table menu in Microsoft Word) to sort the references into alphabetical order. It is important to save the document before you do this in case you do something wrong – you can always revert to your saved version.

Managing a reference list when hand writing an essay

Writing essays by hand is more time consuming than using a computer so you should aim to acquire this IT skill as soon as possible. The easiest way to write a reference list by hand is to write the references on index cards, sort them into alphabetical order as you insert each reference in the text and then write out the list at the end. Alternatively, you could use an indexed (A to Z) notebook and write each reference in the appropriate section. Then you just need to sort each page of references into the correct order before writing them out. Be warned: writing out a reference list by hand is time consuming so allow extra time for this in your planning.

Writing a reference list

There are a number of common errors that students make when writing reference lists. To avoid these:

- Use the designated system correctly (as indicated in your course handbook) and do not mix systems
- Do not number references in the reference list when using the Harvard system
- Do not use first names, just surnames and initials
- Do not use an author's initials or first names in the text, just the surname
- Do not cite an author in the text without including full details in the reference list
- Do not cite unobtainable sources such as your lecture notes

- Punctuate your references correctly (see your course handbook). NB: Books and journals often use an adapted version of the Harvard system, which may be different from that required by your university
- Highlight titles of books and journals correctly.

> **Tip**
>
> Make sure your reference list is correct. Markers will gain an overall impression of your essay from the reference list. They may even look at the reference list before reading the essay. By making sure it is written correctly you will instantly give the marker the impression of competence. Badly written reference lists are often a prelude to a poor or fail grade. Check your handbook for the required referencing system and keep to these guidelines.

Editing your draft essay

Editing is a bit like doing surgery on yourself; it can be painful as it is difficult to discard material that you have spent hours writing. If you find you have exceeded the word limit when you have completed the first draft, try reading your work aloud to identify which sections are too long and boring or repetitive. Ask yourself these questions:

- Can I make the sentences shorter?
- Does this section address the question?
- Will it still make sense if I cut this bit out?
- Have I got too many long quotes that I could shorten by paraphrasing?
- Can I shorten the introduction or conclusion?

Get advice from your personal tutor. Another person's view is likely to be more objective. Just because it's long does not necessarily mean that it's good. Academic work should be comprehensive and concise, hence the word limit.

Save your work regularly

This sounds like stating the obvious but work done on a computer can be lost if not saved regularly. Losing work is frustrating and may put you behind schedule. When working on a computer you must save your work but not just on one disc. Always have a back-up copy as discs can become corrupted and then impossible to use. Writing to CD is a safer option. If it is your own computer, save it to the C drive as well as to two discs (floppy disc or CD) or data or 'memory' stick.

> **Tip**
>
> Get into the habit of saving your work every 10 minutes in case your computer 'crashes'. Yes, this will happen!

Write your conclusion

The essence of a good conclusion is brevity. Do not introduce new ideas; instead make it clear to your reader what you consider to be the key points and emphasise what you feel are the important issues. Keep it short as it may not be allocated a lot of marks. One or two paragraphs should be sufficient. Generally, a good conclusion will add to the overall impression of a well-presented essay (Box 6.4).

Box 6.4 Example of a conclusion

It can be seen that an appreciation of the various sociocultural influences upon a person is vital to understanding how communication can be effective in nursing practice. Nurses need to focus on ensuring that their communications with their patients are unambiguous and contribute to the patients' sense of being cared for sensitively. Maintaining effective communications with members of the multidisciplinary team is also essential to promoting patients' well-being.

Write your introduction

Once you have written the main body you can write the introduction. The purpose of the introduction is to introduce your reader to your essay by outlining the content and the order in which you will discuss issues. This will give your reader a clear framework of the ideas they will encounter in your essay, thus making it easier to follow your arguments. Remember markers will probably have a whole pile of scripts to mark and clarity makes their job much easier. Avoid introducing too much theory in the introduction as this may make it too long but not long enough for you to expand on the ideas. Like the conclusion, not many marks may be allocated to your introduction but it needs to be impressive as it sets the tone of the essay. Avoid long introductions: one clear paragraph should be enough (Box 6.5). If you are writing about your experiences in practice you should include a statement about confidentiality and say that pseudonyms have been used

---

Box 6.5 Example of an introduction

Effective communication is an essential aspect of nursing practice. The aim of this essay is to discuss strategies that nurses can use to improve communication with patients and other members of the multidisciplinary team. Firstly the process of communication will be discussed. Definitions of the terms verbal and non-verbal communication between people will then be explored. Sociocultural aspects, which may affect communication with patients from various groups, will be examined. The possible barriers to effective communication that may occur with patients will be discussed and solutions to these problems will then be considered.

---

instead of patients' real names. The real names of your placement areas should not be used either.

Ask tutors for comments

Ensure your draft is clearly presented with the reference list. Your tutor will not be willing or able to read very rough work. Provide space for comments by leaving good margins and using double line spacing. This could be emailed to your tutor but ensure you have arranged this so that your tutor has time to comment on your work. Tutors may not be prepared to comment on work submitted at the last minute. Be prepared for criticism; that is what will help you to improve. If the feedback indicates that a lot more work is needed then you may need to revise your timetable.

> **Tip**
>
> Do not take criticism of your work personally – it is only your work, not you as a person, which is being criticised. If there are problems with your work it is much better to find out before you submit it.

Write your second draft

If you need to make major revisions in the light of your tutor's comments you should do a new plan. Be careful when 'cutting and pasting' using a computer. If you move sections around ensure you cut out the old section or you may end up with repeated material in your essay, which you may not notice. Again, references need to be checked carefully to ensure any material cited in the text is in the reference list. You should also check that any references deleted from the text during editing are also removed from the reference list.

You may need to further edit this draft if you have too many words. Quotes can be paraphrased to reduce words or you may reduce the length of the introduction and/or the conclusion.

> **Tip**
>
> When saving work on the computer ensure that you save different versions as you may change your mind and go back to an original layout. Put the date in a header or footer or include a version number with the name of the document.

Write your final version of your essay

This is the time to pay attention to detail and make sure there are no typographical errors. It is also a good idea to check your references again, as vital marks can be lost because of sloppy referencing. Once you have finished you might like to print it out on good quality paper, as this will improve the appearance of your work. However, do not be tempted to illustrate your work with a fancy font, florid bullet points or clip art: just keep it plain and simple. Although you may feel fed up with looking at the work at least you can now see the end in sight.

> **Tip**
>
> Do not proofread your work on the computer screen; check a printed version instead using a pencil or pen as a pointer to ensure you check each word carefully. Try to have a break between writing and checking your work.

Hand in your work on time

Use the required folder or binder in which to submit your work according to your university guidelines. Most universities advise you to keep a copy of your work as occasionally things go astray and it is as well to have a back-up. Once it is handed in it is time to stop worrying, as there is nothing more you can do. Relax and have some time off before you start your next piece of work.

> **Tip**
>
> Good essays are never written the night before and if you do there is always the chance a problem may occur with either your computer or printer. Actually, this is just the time when mechanical failures do occur.

Reports and posters

You may be asked to complete assignments in other formats, such as a report or a poster, which again have relevance for your future as a registered nurse. These assignments need to be planned in the same way as essays.

Reports as assignments

Reports are factual accounts with precise details of events. Report writing is an essential nursing skill as records of patient care are legal documents. The process of planning and writing a report is very much the same as for an essay but you will need to structure your report differently, with clearly identified sections and subsections that should be divided with roman numerals or lower case letters to avoid confusion with the pages of your report. You may need appendices (see p. 137) and these should be carefully numbered or labelled with capital letters. A contents list at the front of the report is useful if you have more than two or three appendices.

A clear heading is required for your report stating what it is about. Your report should commence with stated aims and terms of reference, which will indicate the range of issues to be addressed. The first paragraph may contain background information about the subject of the report. The sections will detail events in sequence with clear descriptions. Methods of investigation should be explained and a rationale given for actions, which should include reference to literature or legislation. There should be an analysis of the findings and an indication of proposed actions. Summarise the key points and then draw conclusions from what the report has shown.

Like your essays, the style of writing should be formal; academic and personal opinions should only be included if this is specifically required in the guidelines. If you are asked to comment on an issue in a report, make sure you do not become too personal and, as with essays, be careful with regard to confidentiality if mentioning patients or organisations. You must maintain confidentiality by avoiding improper disclosure of information (NMC 2004).

Producing posters

You may be required to produce a poster for one of your assignments and this is often linked to some form of health education theme. Posters are widely used in community and public health campaigns to promote healthier lifestyles or inform the public and health care workers of innovations or hazards. Poster presentations are also often displayed at conferences and open evenings.

Posters need to be read from a distance of a few feet, so all typed or written material must be large enough to be read clearly. Pictures and slogans are used to catch the viewer's eye. Use colour carefully as some shades, such as pastels, are not easy to read unless on a dark background. The graphics must have a message that is unambiguous and has a clear purpose. Cartoons, symbols and humour must be used with caution as they may not always be cross-cultural and what may seem innocuous to you might be offensive to some viewers. Remember that signs, gestures or nudity, even if it is only a cartoon, may offend some people.

Generally, when creating a poster, simplicity is a good rule as anything too complicated may lessen the impact of your images. It is best to avoid attaching items to a poster, as they may fall off in transit, but if you think this is essential you must check the guidelines to see if it is acceptable. Be careful about using stereotypical images as these may convey an opposite message to that which you intended.

Take advice from others with regard to font style and size. Some styles, though they may look decorative, are not easy to read when you stand back to look at the poster. A plain font such as Arial may be best for text and you should use font size 36 to 78 for key words. You should be able to read the poster at a distance of 1–2 metres.

The layout should be in portrait as this is usually easier to read, and you can enhance the impact with a border of a darker colour to frame the content. Your message should be short but comprehensive; do not be tempted to put too much information on a poster. Leaflets and books are appropriate media for conveying detailed information whereas posters should contain concise advice. You may use 'a play on words' to gain the viewer's attention but again make sure your meaning is clear as not everyone may get the joke or be familiar with English words that have two different meanings (Fig. 6.2).

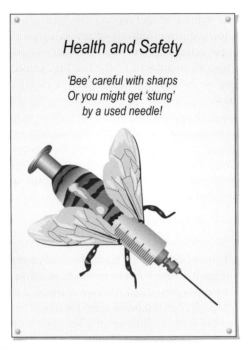

Figure 6.2 Example of a poster

Coping strategies when you are behind with work

Of course it is best to plan ahead and start in good time but in reality you may find that, on occasions, you get behind with assignments. Illness and family commitments can sometimes interfere with your study plans or you may have underestimated how long it would take to complete the assignment or kept putting off starting, thinking the hand-in date was a long way off. If you anticipate that you will not be able to complete an assignment you should seek advice as soon as possible from your personal tutor or module leader.

Seeking an extension

Check the university regulations regarding the policy and procedure for late submissions or extensions, as requests for extensions for your submission are normally only accepted if requested the required number of working days prior to the final submission date. These policies are there to ensure that some students do not have an unfair advantage over other students who have managed to get their work done on time. You must have a very good reason, such as ill health or bereavement, to be granted an extension; poor planning will not usually be considered a good enough reason, neither will problems with a computer or printer. Make sure you allow enough time to make alternative arrangements in the event of computer or printer failure. Seeking an extension may seem like a good idea but remember you will also have the next assignment to start as well.

Getting help from your personal tutor

If there is something affecting your ability to study you should seek help as soon as possible. Your personal tutor may be able to advise you but remember your personal tutor may not be available for last minute help. If you postpone a submission it may mean that you end up with a backlog of assignments. However, if it is a serious problem it is much better to seek an extension or deferral rather than fail your assessment.

You may have to work non-stop for a day to get the assignment finished. Try to avoid too many stimulants such as coffee as these may not keep you going long enough. Non-caffeinated hot drinks and sweets can be good short-term measures. Remember, if you cannot complete your assignment but are too late to request an extension, it is better to submit something and get feedback rather than simply fail because of non-submission.

> **Tip**
>
> When under pressure it is even more important to back up your work by saving on a data/memory stick, floppy disc or CD, as well as your computer's hard drive. Check out alternative places where you can print your essay, as this is the time your printer may fail to work.

Learn from experience

If you achieve a pass grade from an assignment that was a last minute effort you may be persuaded that you work well this way. However, this strategy is unlikely to always be successful. Learn from your experience and plan more realistically in future.

EXAM PREPARATION

You are likely to have exams at some point in your course and these may be written, oral or practical. Written exams come in a variety of formats. You may be told the general subject area (e.g. psychology or ethics) but not the specific topics that you will be tested on; this is usually referred to as an unknown topic exam and you are expected to read widely on the subject. Alternatively, you may be given some information prior to the exam and be expected to research a topic in detail; this is usually referred to as a 'seen topic' or 'known topic' exam.

The way you are required to answer the questions may also vary. The exam may require you to write one long essay, short essays or short answers where a single sentence or word is all that is required, or multiple-choice questions. Sometimes there will be a mixture of multiple-choice and essay questions or short answer questions. Practical exams may be conducted in a skills laboratory or classroom and your performance may be video recorded. Although exams usually last for only a few hours, the preparation required should start weeks if not months beforehand. This preparation involves two important aspects:

● Acquiring the techniques required for specific types of exams
● Revising the subject.

Both are equally important; revising well and using effective exam techniques will certainly increase the likelihood of your passing the exam. Do not leave things to chance. Most universities will offer sessions on exam preparation techniques.

Dealing with exam anxiety

Exams can cause worry, which is actually good as it will motivate you to revise and without this stress you may not bother. However, don't let exam anxiety make you negative. As humans we are physiologically equipped to deal with stressful events and in these instances adrenaline will be released into your blood stream, stimulating you to function more effectively. In an exam this can help you think quickly and recall vital information. So if you feel a bit anxious about an exam it is not an entirely bad thing as you are anticipating a stressful event and your body is responding appropriately. It is natural to have some anxiety related to exams but it is essential that this is managed and contained so that you can effectively use the extra adrenaline circulating in your body, rather than become debilitated by it, as excessive stress can become negative.

Remember that, as a nurse, the ability to function in stressful emergency situations is essential, so it is important that you learn to manage your nerves. Remember that you have been taught to deal with emergencies in clinical practice so focus on what you can do. If you have produced good practice questions when revising then you will be able to answer these in an exam. The thought of exams can be scary but they are never as bad as you might imagine and with confidence can be passed successfully. The key to success is positive thinking and good preparation. If you feel ready for the exam you will not be filled with dread and this will help to prevent you making mistakes.

Stress-reducing techniques

As a nurse you will be advising patients about stress management so it is a good idea to use these health promotion techniques yourself. Excessive stress can be reduced by a number of activities such as breathing exercises, yoga and other relaxation techniques. Check out your local library or health centre for further advice. If you are feeling unwell because of stress, it is appropriate to seek help from your GP, the university health centre or counselling service. Physical exercise of some sort is highly recommended. This does not have to be a strenuous sport; cycling, swimming or simply going for a walk is often as effective for clearing your thoughts and stretching your legs. You should use these activities to break up some of your revision sessions and view them as part of your preparation for the exam.

Avoid negative thinkers

If any of your colleagues continually express negative thoughts about the exam, try to avoid being contaminated by them. It is easy to feel panic if you are exposed to people who overexaggerate the possibility of failure. Remember that you would never have been selected for the course if you did not have the potential to succeed.

Revising for exams

Making a plan or list of all the topics you need to revise is a good idea but you need to be realistic about the actual time you have available and not overestimate the amount of revision you can manage in a week. Try to work steadily for shorter periods rather than long sessions. If you are a morning person you might try getting up an hour earlier, two or three mornings a week, as this is the time when you will most effectively absorb material. You need to review your plan every week and make sure you are achieving your revision targets in the priority subjects.

Getting focused on the subject

Getting focused on exactly what you are supposed to be revising is part of planning your revision. You need to be familiar with the learning outcomes of the relevant section of the course. Check your assignment guidelines or university websites for information. This is an issue that can be discussed in study groups, with your personal tutor and with other lecturers if you are not sure.

Review your notes

Revise your notes and re-write these if you find some areas need more information. Go over lecture notes and underline key points. Make sure you understand all the key points. Check with your timetable and with colleagues in your study group that you have not missed any sessions. The exam will test you on what has been taught.

Make revision cards

Sometimes called flash cards, the aim of revision cards is to reinforce the information in your memory by repeating the information. Reduce your notes to key points on index cards and read these over and over again. You need to start this at least 6 weeks before the exam. The key points should act as triggers to produce a cascade of information when you are in the exam. You can also use these to test each other in a study group.

Make CDs or audio tapes

If you feel that the information is not 'sinking in' when you are reading your notes, it may be that you learn better by auditory means (see 'Learning styles', pp. 33, 34). If so, you may find using the audio method better for reinforcing your notes. When you have re-written your notes, make recordings of these on a tape or CD. These can be played on a portable player as an alternative to visual revision from books and when it is not so easy to read, such as on the bus or out walking.

Practise writing essay questions

You will need to practise planning and answering essay questions. If the exam is to be hand written you must practise writing for the appropriate length of time; this is especially important if you use a computer for much of your work and are no longer used to writing by hand. Practise exam plans and time how long this activity takes. Make a point of obtaining copies of previous exam papers, if these are available; they are usually held in the library, so ask the librarian for help finding them. Alternatively, your personal tutor or course tutor may give you some practice questions to help you revise. This will help you gain confidence for the actual exam. Practising answering questions is best done in three stages.

Stage one

The first stage is the 'perfect answer' stage. This means writing an answer with the help of textbooks and notes. Do not try to answer your question in a set time at this stage. Doing revision in this way in a study group of colleagues can be really helpful.

Stage two

A few days later practise writing the answer again but this time with no textbooks or notes. When you have finished, go back to the books and try to mark your essay. Then think of ways to remember the things you forgot to include in your answer.

Stage three

This is answering a question under exam conditions, i.e. without books or notes and in the allowed time. You need to know exactly how long you will have to answer each question. Writing answers under timed conditions can be best done in the library or quiet study area to avoid distractions. Then you need to get some feedback from your personal tutor or your study group.

Multiple choice questions (MCQ)

In an MCQ test or exam you will be given a question with four or more possible answers and you are required to indicate the correct answer. If you do not know the correct answer you can make a guess, but beware: some multiple-choice exams penalise you if you make the wrong choice. Normally, it will be noted on your instruction paper whether a wrong answer will be given a negative mark. Of the four possible answers, one will usually be clearly wrong. The other three answers may be fairly similar and you will have to determine which one is correct. Because of this you must read each question carefully.

Box 6.6 Example of an MCQ

Select the correct answer from the following:
    The initials NMC stand for which of the following:

- Nursing and Medical Council
- Nursing and Midwifery Council
- Nursing and Medical Corporation
- New Medical Council

You may be asked to complete your exam electronically or manually. Check carefully how to fill in the question paper, as most MCQ exams require you to make a mark in a box beside your selected answer (Box 6.6). An electric scanner is often used to mark these exams so make sure you read the completion instructions carefully.

Tip

Do not spend too long on one question or you may be unable to answer all the questions in the time available. If you are unsure of an answer, move on to the next question and come back to unanswered questions if you have time. Do all the questions you are sure about first.

Short answer exams

Short answer questions (SAQs) usually require single word or short sentence answers so make sure you learn the correct spellings of words that are new to you. Many books include a glossary so check your understanding of definitions of terms as these are often asked for in SAQs. SAQs may also require you to label diagrams, especially if the exam is on a subject such as human biology.

Short essay exams may require a few paragraphs depending on the time allowed. There is often a choice of questions and the paper will state how many of these questions you must answer. Read the instructions carefully. You may only have a few minutes to write an outline plan for your answer but it may be useful to help trigger ideas. Start off with a question that you feel fairly confident about, then tackle the harder ones; however, do not spend too long on one question at the expense of others. As you will probably be required to pass a specified number of questions, you need to divide your time equally and therefore careful timing is essential. If possible, you should allow a few minutes at the end to read through what you have written and make corrections if necessary. Make sure you are clear about how the marks are allocated and what you have to do to achieve an overall pass grade.

Long essay exams

With longer essay exams you may have 1 or 2 hours to answer one question and so will have time to write a more structured answer plan. Write your plan in bullet point form or a diagram (see Fig. 4.10, p. 83); as you cover these points in your answer, tick them off on your plan. When writing your answer you should check at intervals that you are answering the question and not padding out the answer. Be careful to avoid repeating yourself, as this will be evident to the marker.

Leave one or two lines between paragraphs in case you realise you have omitted a vital sentence and need to add it later; this helps to keep the answer neat and legible. Try to pause at regular intervals to check what you have written as it is easy in an exam to repeat material or miss out key words, which can alter the meaning of a sentence. At the end of the exam, cross out any rough work, such as your essay plan, with a single line.

> **Tip**
>
> Don't panic! Remind yourself that you have revised well and know your subject. Be decisive in the exam as panic is fuelled by indecision. Read the question carefully – use your pen as a pointer and read as you move the pen through the sentence and underline key words.
>
> Time management is essential – in short answer exams stop when it is time to move to the next question, as you cannot afford to do well in one question at the expense of others.

Practical exams and vivas

As nursing is a practical profession you are likely to have to some practical exams. These may be in a skills laboratory as Objective Structured Clinical Examinations (OSCEs) or in clinical placements. These require you to perform a number of practical skills using volunteer (simulated) patients or scenarios. A viva (viva voce) requires you to answer a number of oral questions to a small panel of examiners. Although the idea of these types of exam might be a bit nerve-racking, it is important to remember that you are not going to be asked anything you have not been taught and practised in placements with real patients. It has the advantage that you are able to say what you mean rather than having to write it.

Preparing for a viva

In a viva it is important to answer the questions clearly; however, if you find yourself getting into a muddle, just apologise and take a deep breath before beginning again. Try to maintain good eye contact with the examiners and make sure your hands are in a relaxed position on your lap and kept still. Avoid putting your hands in your pockets and fiddling with coins or keys, which can be irritating. Even if you get stuck on a subject try to avoid looking out of a window for inspiration. Never attempt jokes, although your examiners may make a light-hearted comment to put you at ease. Even though you will be anxious to leave the exam it is a good idea to thank the examiners before you leave. Remember you are being assessed as a professional and good interpersonal skills will always create a positive impression.

Preparing for practical exams

These exams put you face to face with your examiner and a confident image is important. As a nurse your patients need to feel that you know what you are doing and can care for them effectively. It is much easier to remain calm when you are confident and so you should use every opportunity to practise and develop your skills. When preparing for practical exams take every opportunity to practise in the skills laboratory. When preparing for a viva it is useful to practise answering oral questions with your colleagues.

On the day, act as if you are looking after a real patient and try to relax. Make sure you have tissues in your pocket if your hands become sweaty. Although chewing gum can help with a dry mouth beforehand, you must dispose of this before you meet your examiners. Pay careful attention to your appearance and ensure if you are in uniform that you are wearing it correctly. You know the importance of non-verbal communication so use it to your advantage by smiling confidently and adopting a poised posture.

When you perform practical skills there is a tendency for your hands to become shaky, especially if you feel nervous because you are being watched. You can over-come this by practising while your fellow students watch. If something does go wrong it does not usually matter as long as you do the right thing to correct the situ-ation, as you would in the clinical area. Take a deep breath and start again. This will demonstrate that you are confident and can deal with the unexpected.

Plans for the day of the exam

Exams are run on very formal lines. If you arrive late you may not be allowed in and this may result in a fail grade. Because of this you must take extra precautions to avoid lateness. At least 2 weeks before, double-check the exam date, time and venue. Plan your route for the day, allowing extra time for travelling. Functioning alarm clocks are necessary and you might like to use the alarm function on your mobile phone as an extra precaution. This might sound excessive but students do sometimes experience problems with oversleeping, especially if they have not slept well because of anxiety. If there is any danger of transport problems (and they are likely to occur), try to have a second plan with an alternative route in mind. Leave plenty of time so that you do not arrive late and make sure you have the necessary documents with you such as identity cards and writing implements. It is now far too late for last minute revision, so avoid it as it will only add to your anxiety and may actually confuse you.

> **Tip**
>
> Check what you are allowed to take into the exam – you will need pens but may also be allowed to take a bottle of drink or sweets to keep away dis-tracting coughs and maintain energy levels. You will not be allowed to have your mobile phone switched on during the exam so make sure you have a watch to keep an eye on the time.

After the exam

It is pointless to advise students to avoid a 'post mortem' discussion after the exam as everyone feels the urge to release the tension by going over the event again. Be warned, however, you may become anxious if you listen to what everyone else said they did and you did not. Some students even convince themselves that they failed to include points when the reverse is true. It is difficult to recall everything you have written or said and trying to work this out may cause unnecessary distress. Try to move on to other things and avoid dwelling on the exam, as this is pointless.

Placement assessments

You will have a number of clinical placements in your programme. The purpose of assessment documents is to provide feedback to your tutors of your performance in practice. A designated practitioner in that area, who has been prepared to undertake this role, will formally assess your performance; this person is often referred to as your mentor. You will be expected to achieve a level of competence, i.e. you will have to show you have learned nursing skills and can apply the theory you have learned in the university campus to the practice environment. The required level of competence in nursing skills will vary according to your stage in the programme. At the beginning of the programme you will be regarded as a novice and will be expected to demonstrate a safe level of performance in a range of fundamental nursing skills under supervision from a registered practitioner. However, by the end of the programme you will be expected to accomplish more complex skills.

Understanding assessment documents

Although your mentor will be familiar with your assessment documents and be able to clarify issues that you do not understand, your mentor will expect you to have read your assessment documents as preparation for your first interview with them in the placement area. Your mentor will discuss with you how you can achieve the required standard of competence and help you devise a learning contract that will state explicitly what you will achieve on the placement and how opportunities to do this will be arranged.

Providing written evidence of learning

Your assessment documents often include a requirement to provide some written evidence to show you have been able to link theory with practice on your placement and the ability to reflect on the knowledge, skills and attitudes that you have acquired during the placement experience. To do this you should keep notes of relevant leaning experiences (ensuring you do not breach confidentiality) and write these up in your reflective journal (see pp. 179, 185).

Linking theory and practice

Your role as a student on placement is to learn through experience but this should be linked to the theory that underpins the actions of nurses. Always think of the reasons for your actions; what distinguishes a professional from a non-professional is the level of underpinning knowledge they have of their work. Increasingly, professionals' practice is examined for effectiveness by the process of audit, which means that nursing decisions must be made in the light of research findings. Make sure that you understand the rationale behind the nursing activities you perform; don't simply do it because 'it has always been done that way'. Using appropriate research findings in practice will ensure that the care given to patients is evidence based. Your performance in practice will integrate your knowledge as well as your psychomotor and communication skills.

Feedback on your performance in practice

You will be assessed on a continuous basis when on placement and should receive both oral and written feedback at specified points of time during your experience. This feedback should indicate how well you are doing and any areas for improvement. Try to develop your skills of self-assessment and make a note of ways in which you consider you have improved or acquired skills as well as areas in need of improvement. This can then be compared to your mentor's assessment of your progress.

Checking your documents

Before leaving your placement area, check that all the assessment documents are completed correctly. Complete any evaluations or feedback forms as required and submit these as directed. You should also, as with other assessments, retain a photocopy.

Self and peer assessment

Self and peer assessment can both be highly effective in helping you improve your performance. It is also an essential part of developing the skills required as a professional nurse. You need to be able to review your performance and determine how you can develop. This means looking not only at *what* you have learned but also *how* you have learned, i.e. not only the product of your learning but also the process. For example, if you did some preparatory reading before attending a lecture you may have then found the new concepts easier to comprehend.

For the process of peer and self-assessment it is necessary to be critical but remember you are using the word criticism in an academic sense, which means judging the positive and negative aspects of something, rather than using criticism in the colloquial sense of only a negative appraisal of a situation. It is usually best to self-assess before asking for feedback from your peers.

Peer assessment as an informal process can occur when you ask fellow students to look at your work and see what they think. The advantage of this is that you can get another person's opinion and make adjustments quickly. In addition, your friends may be able to point out problem areas in your work that you do not see yourself. The disadvantage of this is that the advice you receive may not in fact be helpful. Always remember, just because one of your friends had got through an essay or exam, they may not be able to focus on the weak areas of your work. Also, they may find it hard to give negative feedback because they do not want to hurt your feelings. Always look for a balanced, but honest, view of your work.

Giving and receiving feedback

Peer assessment is part of the process of learning. During activities such as presentations you may be asked to give feedback on your peers' work. In turn you will also experience your fellow students assessing your performance. When giving feedback, start with positive points before moving to areas for improvement. Always give examples when you present a negative point. Be constructive by suggesting alternatives so that a route to improvement is evident. It is important to end on a positive note.

When you are on the receiving end of feedback from peers, try not to be overly defensive; it is about your behaviours, not you as a person. If you feel anxious about the idea of being given verbal feedback in front of other students, you should try to become more aware of your own strengths and weaknesses. This can come from the process of keeping a learning log, which will help you build resilience during times when your work is being criticised in public and sustain your self-belief in your abilities so you can respond positively to suggestions for change.

Things to avoid when giving feedback

- Remember to try to give some positive feedback first. Do not give criticism which is overly destructive. Remember that nursing is a caring profession so do not get carried away when pointing out the deficits in someone's performance.
- Do not spend a disproportional time focusing on negative points that are relatively unimportant. If you mention a small negative point, make it clear that it is just that.
- End your feedback on a positive note but try not to give inappropriate praise just to make the person feel better. This will usually just sound insincere.

Peer assessment is supposed to be a nurturing process so there should be mutual support and all those involved in the activity should be endeavouring to develop new knowledge and skills. Remember that your teachers will also be learning from this process, as they will be assessing their performance as facilitators and looking for improved ways of supporting students' learning.

Using marker's feedback

When you get your work back after marking you will doubtless first look at the mark you have achieved. Many students never get further than this because they are often just relieved to have passed. However, before you file your marked assignments in your portfolio you should read and take note of the written feedback on your work. This is essential so that you can improve next time. As you progress though your course the academic level at which your assignments are judged will be raised. This means that your standard of work must improve. If you have difficulty achieving the required standard or just achieve the pass mark, seek help from academic support services, study skills books and your personal tutor.

> **Tip**
>
> Keep a spreadsheet of your marks as you progress through the course to check that you are improving as you should.

Lack of critical analysis

Critical analysis is a requirement of diploma and degree level work (see Chapter 4) but many students find it hard to achieve. You may receive comments along the lines of 'your work is too descriptive' or 'lacks critical analysis'. This means that your arguments or actions need to be supported by reference to nursing research or concepts that are discussed in nursing literature.

Weak academic style

Markers may note that your work is not written in a good academic style or that you have used informal or colloquial expressions or phrases. Colloquial means using familiar or everyday words as opposed to formal language. This should be avoided because, although the meaning of commonly used phrases may be clear in speech, when they are introduced in the written form ambiguities can occur. Students often make the mistake of writing as if they are talking; you need to adapt your written communication and use an academic style (see Chapter 5).

Limited sources of information

This means that you need to read more about your subject and use a range of information from a variety of books. Sometimes you may find a book that seems to contain all the answers and you can be tempted to look no further for information. However, this will indicate to the marker that you have not looked at alternative views. It is important to remember that just because one author has said that a procedure should be done in a certain way it does not mean that it is the most appropriate way or that it is the most up to date.

> **Tip**
> Do not ignore the feedback, thinking 'it does not matter as long as I have passed'. You may miss vital points that can help to ensure your pass next time.

How to cope with poor marks and failure

Getting poor marks can be depressing, especially if you feel you put a lot of effort into an assignment. You should be given, in your student handbook, some advice with regard to interpreting your mark. Although most universities require a 40% pass mark, you should be aiming for much higher marks. A good grade is normally 70% or above. Less than this indicates some room for improvement and you should be aiming to improve on your next assessment. Your marker will normally give you feedback on your presentation and content of the essay in order to help you improve next time. If they use terms that you do not understand it is important to seek advice from your personal tutor or the marker.

Reasons for failure

Generally, a fail grade means the work is not of a satisfactory standard and usually is awarded for one or more of the following reasons:

- You have not answered the question or not demonstrated the type of knowledge that the assignment is testing.
- Your work was poorly structured, which makes comprehension of your work difficult to follow.
- Incorrect information, faulty referencing or too much irrelevant material.

> **Tip**
>
> Don't get angry if you fail an assessment by a small margin, such as two marks – anything below 40% is significantly less than half right.

Coping with a fail grade

When you get your results and the news is not good there are a number of steps to help you pass when you resubmit your essay or resit your exam.

- It is essential to ask for advice from your personal tutor so arrange an appointment as soon as possible.
- Make a list of the issues that you need to address in your resubmission or exam resit.
- Check the relevant assessment regulations in your student handbook.
- Ensure you make a note of the resubmission or resit date (double check the date).
- Devise a detailed action plan after discussions with your personal tutor and/or specialist subject teacher.
- Ask if there is any support available such as revision sessions or help with assignment writing.

> **Tip**
>
> Be realistic when analysing why you failed. Respond by making a list of the reasons for your failure, not excuses; excuses will not help you to avoid failure next time.

You may feel shocked to have been awarded a fail grade but you must remember it is not you as a person that is a failure, only your work. Take stock of the situation and read the marker's comments again when you have got over the initial disappointment and distress about your result. Then discuss it with the marker if possible, or your personal tutor. Get help with your resubmission but do not rely on friends, even if they have passed the assignment, as they may not be able to give specific advice. A fail grade can be difficult to handle, especially if you feel you did your best. The marker's written feedback should indicate where you went wrong and what you need to do to resubmit your work. Think positively about the event and learn from your mistakes. This way you will be able to approach your resubmission constructively.

Dismiss any idea that teachers want you to fail: this is simply not true. Students often rationalise their bad marks by blaming everyone else. Thinking that your teachers want you to fail could not be more wrong. Remember that teachers want you to pass all your exams and assignments. Your tutors may vary in how they judge your work but any differences between markers are taken into account in a process called moderation. If, after careful consideration, you really do feel that you have been unfairly marked, seek advice from your personal tutor or student representative body. In some universities it is possible to ask for work to be remarked or to appeal against a decision. Most universities will give details of how to do this in student handbooks. Discuss this issue with your personal tutor first.

SUMMARY OF KEY POINTS

- Manage your assignments effectively by planning ahead at all times. Be well organised – it does work.
- Make sure that you understand exactly what is required for all your assessments. If necessary, discuss this with your personal tutor and/or module leader.
- You will cope better with large assignment tasks if you organise them into a series of small manageable tasks.
- Use your personal tutor to help but remember to send your work for comments in good time, as tutors may not always be available to give feedback.
- Be sure to read the feedback from your markers, as this will help you improve next time.
- Exam preparation involves not only revising your subject but also developing the right technique.
- If you do fail an exam or essay, learn from the experience and plan carefully to ensure success next time. Make use of any support that is offered.
- Prepare for practical exams by asking your mentor and colleagues to watch you performing a range of skills; this will help you get used to being watched
- Learn how to give effective feedback to your peers. Be honest; it does not help them if you do not point out areas that need improvement but only mention the good areas.

7

How to learn practical nursing skills

Learning outcomes

This chapter will help you:

- Understand the principles of writing patient records
- Learn how to use your academic writing skills in nursing practice
- Learn psychomotor and practical nursing skills.

Documentation

In nursing, well-written reports and care plans are important not only for continuity of care but also as a legal record of what has happened to the patient during their episode of care. These documents may be read by patients and must be clear and accurate, using appropriate language. Therefore, the ability to write clearly and concisely is as important in nursing practice as it is in your essays and exams.

Patient records

Patient records (also called patient notes) are written about each patient on admission and at the end of every shift or visit and provide a record of the care given. In most clinical areas verbal reports are also given about each patient at the beginning of each shift. This is usually called 'handover' and includes information about the condition of each patient and their treatment, along with other important information, e.g. whether the patient has an infection such as methicillin-resistant *Staphylococcus aureus* (MRSA).

The skills that you develop when writing essays will help you to write patient records that are concise, factual and free from jargon. The Nursing and Midwifery Council (NMC 2004) has issued guidelines for records and record keeping that make clear the legal nature of these documents and the way in which they must be written. According to the NMC (2002b), patient records should be:

- Factual, consistent and accurate, i.e. stating the facts rather than assumptions
- Written as soon as possible after an event has occurred, providing current information on the care and condition of the patient or client
- Written clearly and in such a manner that the text cannot be erased. This means that pencil or erasable ballpoint must not be used
- Written in such a manner that any alterations or additions are dated, timed and signed in such a way that the original entry can still be read clearly. Mistakes should be crossed through with a single line; correction fluid should not be used
- Accurately dated, timed and signed, with the signature printed alongside the first entry. All entries made by student nurses must be countersigned by a registered nurse
- Written without abbreviations, jargon, meaningless phrases, irrelevant speculation and offensive subjective statements
- Readable on any photocopies, which means that records should be written with a black or dark blue pen
- Written, wherever possible, with the involvement of the patient, client or their carer.

Tip

When you are writing reports about the care you have given, remember that these must be countersigned by your supervisor. Ask your supervisor whether they want you to write them together or whether the supervisor will check and sign them later. If they are going to sign them later, make sure you remind them before the end of the shift.

Incident reports

It is also important to make a record of any unexpected incident that occurs, e.g. incidents such as a patient falling out of bed or a medication error. When writing a statement for an incident form it is important to be completely factual and to avoid making any assumptions; you must state only what you know to be true and what you actually observed. For instance, if writing about a patient who fell, it is not your role to make assumptions about what other staff were doing; you must state only what *you* were doing and what you observed other staff to be doing (e.g. 'I saw staff nurse Jones standing by the ward door' rather than 'Staff nurse Jones was checking whether the patient was in the ward or outside'). The use of correct terminology and attention to detail is essential, e.g. whether the lights were switched on or whether the floor was dry.

Identification bands

Although you may not consider these to be documents, they are written communications which, if completed incorrectly, could have serious consequences. Identification (ID) bands (also called name bands) are used in institutional settings as patients may not be able to identify themselves if they are either unconscious or unable to speak. They require neat, clear writing in a small space. Make sure your letters and numbers are clearly distinguishable, e.g. the number '1' and the letter 'I' can be mistaken. When writing the data on an ID band, careful checking of details is essential to ensure that they correspond with those in the medical notes. ID bands should have the full name, date of birth and hospital registration number (NB: make sure similar numbers such as 1 and 7 and 3 and 5 are clear). The name of the ward is sometimes included.

Charting

Charting the results of clinical observations is a routine part of most nurses' practice. In some areas results will be written in the care plan or patient notes but in most acute settings they will be written on a chart. The whole point of using charts is to make it easy to see trends, i.e. whether the patient's vital signs are stable, getting better or getting worse. For this reason it is important to chart your results accurately and neatly; untidy charts make it difficult to identify any problems. Figure 7.1 illustrates two charts that include exactly the same information but, as you can see, the chart in Figure 7.1a clearly shows what is happening to the patient's temperature, pulse and respiration rate whereas on the chart in Figure 7.1b it appears that the temperature and pulse rate are going up and down in an erratic fashion.

> **Tip**
>
> Always check that the patient's details are written at the top of the chart before entering any observations and never chart observations on a chart with no name. This could be confusing and potentially dangerous as it may be assumed to belong to a different patient.

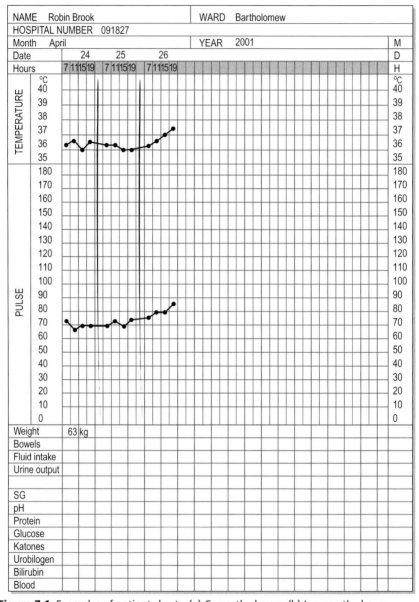

Figure 7.1 Examples of patient charts. (a) Correctly drawn. (b) Incorrectly drawn.

Clinical charts should be considered as mathematical graphs designed to show trends in the observations that you are recording. This means that you need to use agreed symbols for the recording; a dot is usual for temperature, pulse and respiration rate and an 'x' or inverted 'v' (∧) with a dotted line joining the two marks for blood pressure. Recordings should be joined with a straight line as shown in

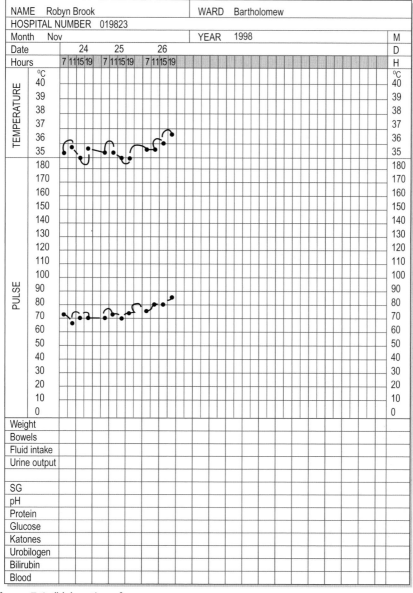

NAME	Robyn Brook												WARD	Bartholomew																	

HOSPITAL NUMBER   019823

Month   Nov — YEAR   1998 — M

Date: 24, 25, 26 — D

Hours: 7 11 15 19   7 11 15 19   7 11 15 19 — H

TEMPERATURE (°C): 40, 39, 38, 37, 36, 35

PULSE: 180, 170, 160, 150, 140, 130, 120, 110, 100, 90, 80, 70, 60, 50, 40, 30, 20, 10, 0

Weight
Bowels
Fluid intake
Urine output

SG
pH
Protein
Glucose
Katones
Urobilogen
Bilirubin
Blood

Figure 7.1 (b) (*continued*)

Figure 7.1a; curved lines (often referred to as tadpoles!) must not be used as they distort the picture and make it difficult to identify trends. In some clinical areas it is common practice to write the figures next to the systolic and diastolic blood pressure recordings. This should not be necessary if they are charted accurately and can make the chart cluttered and difficult to read; however, if that is the way it is done in your placement area you should do the same, writing the figures neatly to prevent obscuring the chart.

> **Tip**
>
> In your placements you will come across a variety of symbols and ways of charting observations. Most nurses have their preferred way of doing this but when entering recordings on a chart it is best to insert your observations in the same way as the previous person (e.g. using an 'x' or 'ʌ') as this makes it clearer and easier to read.

Electronic patient records

It is now increasingly common for patient's notes to be computerised. In the future it is likely that nearly all notes will be electronic. Therefore it is essential for nurses to be computer literate, and you should use every opportunity, such as completing essays and other assignments, to use a computer and improve your skills. If at university in the UK it is likely that you will be required to achieve the European Computer Driving Licence (www.ecdl.com) qualification (see also Chapter 3).

LEARNING PRACTICAL SKILLS

During your programme you will be learning a wide range of practical skills. Learning practical skills is often thought to be easier than learning facts and theories. In fact, learning practical skills is not simply a matter of copying what your lecturer does, it is important that you understand not only what to do but also why you are doing it, how you are doing it and the underlying theoretical principles. Bloom (1956) described three domains of learning: the cognitive domain (mental skills or knowledge), the affective domain (feelings, emotions and attitudes) and the psychomotor domain, which refers to manual skills. All three domains are involved when learning to be a nurse but in this section we will focus on acquisition of psychomotor skills and how to prepare for the practical exams and assessments that are likely to be a part of your programme.

Learning psychomotor skills

Psychomotor skills are an important part of nursing; however, unlike other forms of learning, they require practice, i.e. repetition of a procedure in order to be learned. This is because it takes time to learn and produce skilled, efficient movement (Quinn 2000). Fitts and Posner (1967) described three phases that occur during skill acquisition: the cognitive phase, the associative phase and the autonomous phase.

The cognitive phase

In this phase you identify the component parts of the skill and then form a mental picture of the skill. This phase is concerned with learning the procedure: the more complex the skill, the longer this will take (Quinn 2000). For example, correctly remembering each stage of the procedure for blood pressure (BP) measurement will take longer than learning the procedure for weighing a patient. It is important to try to understand why each step of the procedure is necessary rather than merely copying what has been demonstrated.

When learning a new skill, first observe the skill all the way through without interruption. Watch carefully and try not to let your mind wander onto other things. Then write down what you observed. If you are doing this on your placement it may not be feasible to do it straight away. You should, however, do it as soon as possible while the procedure is still fresh in your mind. By making yourself remember each stage you will be imagining the procedure in your mind. Writing down each step in sequence will help you to commit the procedure to memory.

Having imagined yourself performing the skill it is important to perform the procedure yourself, using your notes for guidance or, if on placement, under supervision. When you have performed the skill at least once you will know how it feels and will then be able to use a technique called mental rehearsal to maintain and improve your level of skill.

Mental rehearsal

Mental rehearsal means the mental practice of performing a skill as opposed to actual practice. When engaging in mental rehearsal you imagine performing an activity without actually doing anything (Williams 2005). This means more than simply thinking about a procedure; it means imagining that you are actually performing that procedure and feeling, seeing, hearing (and even smelling if appropriate!) as you would if you were actually doing it. This technique is most useful when you have developed a reasonable level of skill because you are then able to rehearse good performance. It can also help you to cope with the stress of practical exams and assessments because mental practice improves self-confidence and you can reduce your stress levels by visualising yourself performing well in your exam.

To perform the mental rehearsal technique (based on Williams 2005):

1. Find a time when you will not be interrupted.
2. Close your eyes, relax and focus.
3. Tell yourself that you are confident and have the ability to perform this procedure well. Repeatedly tell yourself, with confidence, that you will be successful.
4. Mentally picture yourself just before you start the procedure or begin the exam – make sure you stay relaxed and focused.
5. Now mentally rehearse successful performance of the skill. Make sure you imagine yourself actively performing the skill, not just watching. For example, if mentally rehearsing BP measurement, imagine sitting by the bed, touching the BP cuff and placing it around the patient's arm. Imagine the feel of the brachial pulse as you check its position. Imagine every step of the procedure, including hearing the BP and writing it on the chart.

6. Now open your eyes and smile. You have successfully performed BP measurement and should now be confident that you will perform successfully in the real situation. Praise yourself for being successful – praising yourself is helpful because self-reinforcement is a key to self-motivation.

Mental rehearsal can be a useful technique because you may not always be able to practise physically and maintain all the skills you need. This may be because some procedures do not occur in your placement or, when not on clinical placement, you may not have access to the equipment that you need. Mental rehearsal can help you to maintain and improve your level of skill when physical rehearsal is not possible, boost your self-confidence and help you cope with the stress of practical exams and other assessments.

The associative phase

The associative phase is when your performance has become skilled and mistakes or omissions have been eliminated. In this phase your performance is accurate but you still need to think carefully about each step of the procedure. This is sometimes called 'conscious competence' (Howell & Fleishman 1982).

The autonomous phase

The autonomous phase is when the psychomotor aspects of the skill have become automatic and can be performed without thinking about it. This is also known as 'unconscious competence' which means that you no longer have to concentrate on each step and you can do it while your mind is on other things. For example, you are no longer conscious of *how* you write; you are free to concentrate on *what* you are writing. Once you no longer need to concentrate on *how* to perform BP measurement you are free to concentrate on other things such as communicating with the patient, promoting patient comfort, factors that might affect the BP and whether the reading is normal.

Practice makes perfect

The length of time that it takes to learn a practical skill will vary and most people can identify at least one practical skill that took them ages to learn. So if it seems to be taking you longer than others to master something, do not despair; it just means that you need more practice than they do for that particular skill. Most universities and many hospitals will have practical rooms or skills laboratories where you can go to practise. You will probably have to book, so check out the procedure and relevant phone numbers, etc. With a lot of nursing skills you will need someone to act as your patient, so get a small group of three or four of you together so that you can all practise on each other.

When to practise

You will probably be able to perform a lot of practical skills on your clinical placements but performing a procedure on a real patient for the first time can be quite daunting if you are unsure of yourself and don't feel very confident. Practising in a skills laboratory will improve your confidence and when able to use these skills

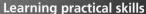

with real patients your confidence will soar. The patients and the nurses who are supervising you will also give you feedback to help you perfect your skills.

> **Tip**
>
> When practising in the skills laboratory, create your own checklist of the procedure and ask your friends to watch you and give you feedback. Then swap and do the same for them. Remember to give each other positive feedback first, i.e. identify what they did well, before you tell them what they need to improve. It is important to be honest.

Distributed practice, i.e. practice sessions separated by rest periods or longer periods of time (e.g. days), is more effective than massed practice, i.e. practising over and over again for hours on end without rest (Quinn 2000). Distributed practice avoids boredom, fatigue or loss of concentration. You need to be motivated for any period of practice so it is better to plan several short practice sessions rather than trying to cram in all your practice on the day before the exam. Not only is it not likely to be effective, you will probably find the skills laboratories very busy and have difficulty getting in.

Objective Structured Clinical Exams (OSCEs)

The OSCE is a form of practical exam that is gaining increasing popularity in nursing and other health care professions. There are a number of different formats but all will involve testing your ability to perform a range of practical procedures in front of an examiner, usually one of your lecturers (Harden & Gleeson 1979). You may be required to demonstrate competence in a practical procedure using a model or manikin (e.g. injections) or with a volunteer (simulated) patient. The assessor will mark your performance against an agreed checklist.

Being watched is always a little daunting and will make you conscious of your every move and action. It is important to feel confident about the skills that will be tested and practising with others watching you is good preparation and will help you get used to the idea.

> **Tip**
>
> When demonstrating a procedure in an OSCE, imagine that the assessor is the nurse who is supervising you on the ward. Imagine that it is someone that you enjoyed working with and who gave you support and confidence to do well.

OSCE checklists

Most OSCE examiners use agreed checklists that detail the procedure for the various skills. If you have copies of these in advance of the OSCE it is important to recognise that they are merely checklists and therefore only useful for self-assessment, not learning. They will, of course, help you identify the key stages of each procedure but it is important not to simply memorise the checklist; memorising the checklist will lead to superficial learning and will prevent you really understanding what you are doing and why. In addition, your memory may let you down when under stress during the OSCE.

However, memory techniques (e.g. mnemonics, see p. 24) can be useful for helping you to remember key safety or accuracy points. For example, most nurses are familiar with the AAAA, B and C of resuscitation. The four As (Approach, Assess, Assistance and Airway) are triggers to help you remember to: Approach the casualty with caution to ensure that you are not putting yourself in danger; Assess the casualty's level of consciousness by speaking loudly in both ears and gently shaking their shoulder, etc. (Nicol et al 2004). Creating your own stories or mnemonics to help you remember key things is a good idea (see p. 26).

Learning while on clinical placement

Your clinical placements will be designed to help you develop a whole range of practical skills and the clinical staff are there to help you. You will probably have some kind of assessment document (e.g. Skills Schedule) which lists all the skills that you have to achieve before entry to the Branch Programme at the beginning of the second year, and others that you have to achieve before entry to the Professional Register at the end of your 3-year programme (NMC 2004).

Once you have had time to settle into your placement and have a good idea about the sort of nursing activities that occur there, go through your list of skills and identify which ones you should be able to achieve in that placement. Then divide them up into those that can be achieved straightaway and those that would be better left until later in your placement. Try to focus on practising at least one skill per shift. Plan the day before and at the beginning of the shift tell your supervisor which skill(s) you would like to achieve. It is best to do this before the patients have been allocated so that your supervisor can ensure that you are allocated to appropriate activities that will enable you to achieve your skills. For example, if you identified that you wanted to develop your moving and handling skills your supervisor will be able to make sure that you are involved in the care of dependent patients rather than those who are fully mobile.

Supervision

Remember that you must be supervised by a registered nurse at all times. There are two types of supervision: direct and indirect.

Direct supervision

Direct supervision means that your supervisor can see what you are doing. This means that the supervisor must be close at hand so that they can quickly intervene if necessary. As a student nurse you are only allowed to be involved in the administration of medicines (including nebulisers and intravenous infusions) under the *direct supervision* of a registered nurse, regardless of your level of competence. This is because only registered nurses are able to administer medicines. However, with other skills, once you have demonstrated that you are competent to perform them alone, you will work under indirect supervision.

Indirect supervision

Indirect supervision means that you are not always being observed directly by the registered nurse; however, the RN is acting as a resource when you need help and is accountable for the care that you provide under their supervision. Indirect supervision means that you may perform aspects of care on your own (e.g. clinical observations or urinalysis) but will then inform your supervisor about the results and any abnormal findings.

Tip

When you are reporting a patient's observations (temperature, pulse, respiration rate and blood pressure) to your supervisor, try to anticipate what your supervisor will say or do. For example, if your patient's blood pressure is rather low and their pulse rate is raised, what might be causing this? Think back to your biology sessions and try to work out what affects blood pressure and the rationale for the action that your supervisor takes. If you are lucky, your supervisors and other healthcare professionals (e.g. doctors, physiotherapists) will 'think aloud' as they work so that you can understand the reasoning that underpins their action.

Making known your limitations

The NMC *Code of Professional Conduct* (NMC 2004) requires you to inform an appropriate person if you are not competent to perform a particular skill or procedure and emphasises that you must not perform any nursing activity unless competent to do so. This means that you must not attempt any nursing activity without first having been taught how to do it. That teaching may be in the university or in clinical placement and does not have to be a formal teaching session; however, if you have not been taught the skill in the university it is important to inform your supervisor. This is because if you have had no previous teaching your supervisor will have to act as both teacher and supervisor to ensure that you understand the underlying rationale and underpinning theories as well as demonstrating the procedure.

As a student nurse it is your responsibility to ensure that you do not attempt any activity for which you have not received adequate training. In busy clinical placements it is tempting to try to help hard-worked staff by 'having a go' at skills you have never done before, without proper supervision and teaching. However tempting, you *must never* perform any nursing activity alone until you have been assessed as competent to do so. It can sometimes feel awkward having to explain that you are unable to do something, particularly when that skill is something that the nurses assume you are able to do. One way to deal with this is to say: 'I'm sorry, I've not been taught to do that. Can I watch you this time then I'll be able to do it next time with you watching me.' A response like that will demonstrate that you are keen to learn and are taking your responsibilities seriously. It is your responsibility to ensure that you have the necessary competence before accepting any delegated duty.

SUMMARY OF KEY POINTS

- Improving your essay writing skills will help you to write good patient records and care plans.
- Mental rehearsal of practical skills can help you to maintain your skills when not in clinical placements.
- Asking your friends to watch you and give feedback on your performance can help you prepare for practical exams (OSCEs).
- Using memory techniques such as mnemonics can help you remember key safety or accuracy points.
- Charting clinical observations is an important nursing skill. Charts should be treated as mathematical graphs and filled in neatly to enable trends to be detected.
- When on clinical placement you must be supervised by a registered nurse at all times and it is your responsibility to ensure that you do not attempt any activity for which you have not received adequate training.

8

How to learn from experience: becoming a reflective practitioner

Learning outcomes

This chapter will help you learn how to:

- Prepare your professional portfolio
- Develop a reflective approach to your learning
- Keep a reflective diary or journal
- Prepare a learning contract.

PORTFOLIOS

A portfolio is a systematic, purposeful and meaningful collection of a student's work in one or more subject areas (DeFina 1992). A curriculum vitae (CV) provides a résumé of a professional's qualifications and experience whereas a portfolio can demonstrate in a more detailed way a person's knowledge and skills.

Your portfolio

Many professionals who need to sell their services, e.g. architects, artists and models, have long used portfolios to showcase their past work. Your portfolio should be a detailed, formal collection and record of your learning experiences (Fig. 8.1). This can be used for assessment purposes or for a general account of continuing professional development. A portfolio can also be more than this; it can be used to stimulate learning. For example you can use it to examine the profile of your educational achievements and you may see areas for further development. You might like to include in your portfolio your short- and long-term career objectives. Having written plans can help you identify what you need to study next. As a student, your portfolio should provide the evidence that demonstrates your ability to meet the outcomes and standards laid down by the NMC.

> ### Tip
>
> Check the programme outcomes or objectives in your course materials to help you visualise what you should have achieved at the end of the course and what is needed in your portfolio to demonstrate this learning. For example, the ability to plan patient care can be demonstrated by a nursing care plan you have written for an assignment.

Throughout your course your portfolio will be the record of your achievement of your learning outcomes, both in the university campus and in placement areas. It is your responsibility, as an adult learner, to keep your portfolio up to date. Recording your learning activities to create a profile of you as a registered practitioner is a good habit to acquire and will help you plan your future learning throughout your career. Your university will keep a record of your progress as a student but this will remain with the university. Your portfolio is your personal property and therefore yours to keep. You may need to present your portfolio at the end of your programme and you will require a portfolio of your knowledge and skills as a registered nurse.

Lifelong learning and portfolios

If you are wondering why you should have to keep records of your learning, think about what you would expect of a registered nurse. A nurse who has experience and is up to date is likely to figure highly in your expectations. This is also the

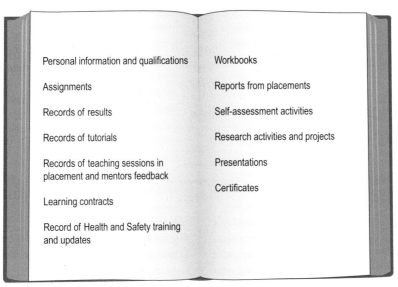

Personal information and qualifications	Workbooks
Assignments	Reports from placements
Records of results	Self-assessment activities
Records of tutorials	Research activities and projects
Records of teaching sessions in placement and mentors feedback	Presentations
	Certificates
Learning contracts	
Record of Health and Safety training and updates	

Figure 8.1 Example of a portfolio

expectation of the Nursing and Midwifery Council (NMC) which requires the following:

> *You must keep your knowledge and skills up to date throughout your working life. In particular you should take part regularly in learning activities that develop your competence and performance.*

(NMC 2004: 9)

This is what a portfolio would demonstrate and employers need clear records, not only of a nurse's qualifications, but also evidence that there has been continuing education and development to improve old skills and learn new ones. The NMC requires all registered nurses to maintain an up-to-date portfolio. Keeping a portfolio demonstrates a commitment to learning that should continue throughout your professional life.

How should a portfolio be presented?

The presentation of your portfolio should indicate that you are well organised so spend time on making a good impression by arranging your work in a logical order with a clear contents page at the beginning. Your portfolio items will need to be arranged as a collection and this can be a file, which you have divided into sections, or you may wish to purchase a commercially produced portfolio. Your university may provide some documents for your portfolio and guidelines as to how it should be compiled. The essential thing is that you start working on your portfolio at the outset, with a clear system for putting your portfolio items in order.

The contents of your portfolio

Your portfolio should contain items which demonstrate your knowledge and skills, such as essays, exam feedback documents, reports from placement and mentors' comments, self-assessment documents and learning contracts from placement, and copies of attendance records or timesheets.

You may also include records of training in relation to Health and Safety, Manual Handling, Fire Safety, First Aid, Resuscitation and periodic updates of these and any certificates of attendance at other training sessions that you attended while on placement. You will need to keep records of when you have undergone updating activities for these procedures as a student and as a registered nurse. You should also keep brief records of supervision meetings with your personal tutor and placement records.

Tip

Try to make time to update your portfolio at the end of a term or module on a regular basis. This is an excellent practice to instigate for the rest of your career as a nurse. For example, when you get an essay returned to you this should be filed directly in your portfolio.

Material or items which should not be placed in a portfolio

Be careful: *do not* include in your portfolio inappropriate documents, as follows:

- Confidential information – you must exclude any item which breaches patient confidentiality. Patients must never be named or in any other way identified.
- Blank forms, charts or any other form of documentation, which are the property of a health care trust or other organisation, must not be used as this does not demonstrate learning and wastes resources. Do not be tempted to try to 'pad out' your portfolio.
- You must never take photocopies of patient notes. These legally belong to the health care trust.
- If you ever wish to include photographs of placement areas, either in assignments or your portfolio, appropriate permission from a manager must be obtained in writing.

Developing your portfolio

As you progress through your course you should regularly review your portfolio. Rather than just filing items, make a point of looking for evidence of your own development. For assignments such as exams and essays compare marks to see if you are improving or can identify areas to develop. Try to analyse the feedback from markers to identify areas where you still need to develop, e.g. check to see if you have made the same errors on more than one occasion. Do not be dismissive of poor marks: be objective and learn from your mistakes. On the other hand, you need to recognise where you have done well.

Another area for review could be your placement learning contracts and mentors' feedback. Is there a similarity of comments from your various mentors? Are

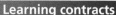

there issues you need to address in your practice and are you setting yourself realistic objectives? Have you enjoyed your placements, and if not why? Do you feel confident that you can easily obtain pass grades in your practice placement assignments? If so, you may identify areas where you need to set yourself tougher challenges to achieve a higher level of skills.

Overall, your review of your placements should not only be a balance of recognising achievements and praising yourself but also being aware of where you need to develop and how you can address your future learning needs in your next learning contract.

LEARNING CONTRACTS

An expectation of university students is that they are self-directed and learning contracts can help to foster the skills of self-directedness (Knowles 1986). This means that, as a student, you are expected to determine what your personal learning needs are and to be proactive in making arrangements to meet your needs. This can help you to be an active rather than a passive learner. Instead of being told exactly what you will learn, you can say what you would like to learn. You might initially feel unsure about this requirement to be active in your learning. However, once you get used to the process you will reap the rewards of feeling in control of your learning experiences. Rolfe et al (2001) consider that learning contracts are an effective basis for lifelong learning to help practitioners achieve career goals.

A contract is an agreement that specifies terms and conditions. A learning contract is a formal written agreement between learner and supervisor which should denote the exact expectations of learning that should occur in the period of learning to which it relates. As a student you have a responsibility to make use of learning opportunities and registered nurses have a professional responsibility to facilitate the gaining of competence by student nurses and midwives (NMC 2004). These obligations underpin your learning contract, which should be agreed when you commence a placement.

Preparing a learning contract

Central to a learning contract are clearly stated objectives and assigned responsibilities. Therefore you should be prepared to state what you wish to learn and your supervisor or mentor will agree if these are appropriate and achievable. Preparation of your personal learning objectives will link to the stated learning outcomes in your programme handbooks. So find out what it is you are expected to learn and merge these with your own learning needs. It is therefore a good idea to draft your requirements prior to the meeting when your learning contract will be agreed.

Self-assessment is the key to determining what you need to learn and this may come from feedback from previous supervisors or mentors. This means that you need to be prepared to look objectively at the feedback you are given and analyse where further development is required. You might consider what skills, knowledge and attitudes you have to develop. These must be realistic in that, for example, you should ensure you are competent at key skills such as observation, communication and providing safe physical care before trying to obtain complex skills. Listen carefully to suggestions from your supervisor or mentor, as they will have more insight with regard to the potential learning experiences that are available and desirable according to your level of competence.

There is also a difference in the level of expertise that may be acquired with what you may consider are basic skills such as taking pulses. This means that you may still have to practise skills to become more proficient, even if at one stage you have achieved a safe level of practice. As you progress through your programme, staff in placement areas will have higher expectations of your performance and for this reason you should always be prepared to improve even basic skills.

How your learning contract will be used for assessment

Your learning contract will be reviewed at various times during and at the end of the learning experience to determine what has been achieved. This assessment will also focus on how you have contributed to your learning with regard to motivation and enthusiasm. The review will allow you to consider what should be incorporated into the next learning contract and help you to further develop as a self-directed student.

What is a reflective practitioner?

You should aspire to become a reflective practitioner. This term implies that the practitioner functions in the context of frequently examining their performance and adjusting their actions in the light of learning from experience. This sounds like stating the obvious but reflection should be in some way formalised and recorded to obtain maximum benefit from the process of self-examination. This means making written accounts of events and reviewing these in a systematic way, which has a constructive purpose that does not focus on blame but on learning.

The regularity of the review process can be variable and the degree or intensity of the reflections can be in proportion to the complexity of the experience. For students on a short placement of 1–2 weeks it might be beneficial to reflect every day or two, but this level of activity is perhaps unrealistic on a longer placement such as one lasting 10–12 weeks. It has to be undertaken when the individual is not overly physically tired or concerned with family responsibilities. However, it is an activity that should be planned for during placement at some appropriate time. It can be undertaken individually or in a study group, which can be especially helpful when attempting to see issues from alternative viewpoints.

A reflective practitioner is one who is always open to the idea of reviewing their performance and being prepared to make changes, however small, to their practice in the light of these considerations. Although it can be difficult to accept criticism, it can be easier if you learn not to take this as focused on you as a person but more on behaviour that has to be adjusted in the future. However, if you are not able to take criticism this may become a barrier to reflection. Self-assessment should take the form of giving feedback to yourself – you should first consider positive aspects of your performance. Then try to be objective about your behaviour and actions and attitudes. Try to avoid being over-critical, which may make you focus on yourself as a failure, as it is unlikely that all your behaviour or intentions are wholly remiss.

REFLECTION AND REFLECTIVE JOURNALS

Learning from experience is the fundamental way in which humans learn. Recognising all that we have learned from a particular experience requires a bit more thought, and trying to relate that experience to theory and even develop theory from the experience can be a little more challenging! Nursing is a practical activity and thus nurses can learn by 'doing' or from their experiences. Nurses as professionals need to be reflective in order to review and learn from their experiences. This skill will enable you to continue to develop throughout your career. Completion of training is not the end point of learning for nurses: there never is an end point for acquiring knowledge, skills or attitudes of how to deal with nursing situations.

What is reflection?

There are different uses of the term reflection. It can mean seeing an image that is visible in a glass or mirror or it can be concerned with a mental process of looking back at events and thinking about them in a different way. It is this second meaning that is the basis of reflection as a skill. When deciding what reflection is about, it might be helpful if you try to think of other terms for this activity of being reflective, such as consideration, deliberation, musing, being pensive, introspection, meditation and contemplation. What these have in common is that they involve thinking more deeply, with a questioning or analytical approach, about issues or experiences.

Why is this important?

Professionals are answerable for their practice and they must ensure through self-analysis that their practice is appropriate and current. In the ever-changing world of nursing you need to be aware of how and what you have learned from new experiences. Through reflection you will be examining actions in a systematic manner and this will enable you to identify effective and non-effective behaviours. Learning skills related to self-development equip you to cope with new and difficult situations that may arise when you assume greater responsibility as a registered nurse. Your pre-registration programme is preparing you for your lifetime as a professional, i.e. one who will be required to be continually updated. Continuing professional development is about evolving skills, knowledge and attitudes in a creative and proactive manner to ensure your qualification is fit for the area in which you practise.

Starting to reflect

If you are feeling hesitant about the process of reflection, try doing this in a staged approach. There are frameworks for reflection but, as a first step – especially if you are not sure exactly 'what it is you are reflecting about' – start by writing a description of an event and then ask yourself some questions about the practice:

- Was it legal?
- Was it ethical?

- Was it professional?
- Was it safe?
- Was it technically correct?
- Was it based on current evidence-based practice?
- Was it organised or managed in an efficient manner?

From this initial material you can reconsider the event in the light of nursing theory. This is where you check out responses and actions with what you could or should have done according to the views of experts. You then might start to formulate some alternatives if things could have been done differently. Alternatively, considering the possible theoretical basis for your actions may confirm that appropriate actions were in fact taken. It is important that you recognise achievements as well as identifying areas for future development.

Writing reflectively

Your tutors want you to demonstrate that you have the ability to learn from your experiences. It is important to recognise where your practice was effective so that you are aware of your strengths and can build on these as well as develop in areas where you have some weaknesses. If you are new to this idea of reflection and feel a bit lost by the requirement to write reflectively, don't worry. It is a skill that you just need to practise and develop. You should to learn to analyse your practice and prepare action plans to develop areas where you are deficient in a positive way. When you reflect you can think about the event generally and try to analyse your learning, or you might like to use a tool such as a reflective framework. You do not have to use a framework (see 'Using a reflective framework', below) but you may find that this enables you to reflect more effectively (see Boxes 8.1, 8.2).

Sometimes it is difficult to 'get started'. However, if you maintain a diary during your practice you will find that you will remember events more clearly. From your diary (see 'Keeping a reflective diary or journal', below) you should be able to draw out events or experiences that seemed, at the time, significant to you. This experience may be something that you did, a training session that you attended or events that you witnessed. Start by breaking down an event or experience into sections that relate to and describe different activities and, if applicable, what the people in the event were actually doing. The process of thinking about the component parts of an event will help you when you start to analyse the experience.

For example, if I was reflecting on a lecture that I have given I may think about this event in terms of preparation, introduction, middle, conclusions, resources and questions asked by students. In a practice situation you may think of an event in terms of the part you played, the part the patient/client played and the role that other health care professionals played. Alternatively, you could take an approached based more on the chronology of an event such as preparation to deliver care, initiation of patient contact, delivery of care, evaluation of immediate impact and leaving the patient. There is no correct way to break down the description of an event; it just helps when it comes to analysis. When you are describing the event for others, say as part of an assignment, you may simply recall the event as a narrative;

however, it is still a good idea to break down the description even if you do not reveal that description to anyone else.

Reflection can also be helped if you initially outline what you think you have learned. You may want to break this down into types of learning, such as:

- Knowledge/understanding
- Skills
- Values and attitudes.

For each you may like to think of Rudyard Kipling's five verities of man: where, who, what, when and why. Thinking in this way will help you to identify what your experience was and what you learned from it. Sometimes it helps to conduct these preliminary phases working with a colleague or friend. After describing the event, probably as you would a story (narrative), you may now want to consider your feelings and emotions. What were your emotions (e.g. compassion, anger, fear, warmth) and why do you think you had those emotions? Having conducted the preliminaries you can now move to using a more structured approach by selecting a reflective model.

Using a reflective framework

Reflection involves examining personal experiences through discussion, either written or orally. As a process it is not necessarily bound by rigid conventions but nevertheless it should have a structured approach and at all times respect information that is confidential in nature. Using a reflective framework can help to direct the writer to move from description towards analysis. This enables you to reframe and reinterpret experiences so that they can be examined in the light of theoretical knowledge.

There are several models or frameworks that are available to help us use reflection. Two very popular models are those of Johns (1992) and Gibbs (1988). Johns's model is linear in its nature whereas Gibbs's model (Fig. 8.2) is always described

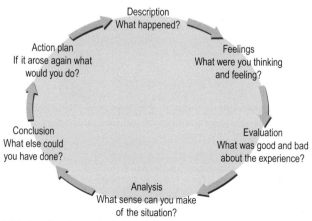

Figure 8.2 Gibbs's reflective cycle (after Gibbs 1988)

Box 8.1 Example of reflection using the Gibbs cycle (Gibbs 1988)

Description

I did not do well in my exam. In fact I failed the exam. However, I did not use the time for independent study to do extensive revision but I did do some revision.

Feelings

What were you thinking and feeling? At first I was shocked to find I had failed and felt we should have been given more support. I did not think I had been marked fairly and was very angry to have failed by a few marks. After a while I felt angry with myself that I had let everyone down.

Evaluation

What was good and bad about the experience? This was a bad experience for me and at first I could not see anything that was helpful in my situation, rather that everyone was against me. However, what was good in retrospect is that it made me realise that I should use my time well and if I failed it was my own fault. I had simply not studied when given days off to do so and instead used the time for other things, thinking I would catch up later. I should have worked on my studies.

Conclusion

What else could you have done? I could have taken a more proactive approach and organised my study days and not relied on the fact that having recently done an access course I would be able to pass.

Analysis

What sense can you make of the situation? I had thought I was a self-directed learner but examining my approach to study days I think I was somewhat resistant to the idea. Brookfield (1986) notes that learners should be eased into this mode of study. However, although we were encouraged to see ourselves as adult learners, clearly I needed more guidance or the experience of failure to change my behaviour.

Action plan

If it arose again, would you do it again? I have a new approach to my studies and plan ahead. I do not even think about calling a study day a day off. I would also advise other students to be much more serious, even if they think they know the subject, in working hard for exams.

Box 8.2 Johns's (1992) model of reflection

Core question: What information do I need to access in order to learn through this experience?

1. Description of the experience:
   - Phenomenon – What is the 'here and now' experience?
   - Causal – What essential factors contributed to this experience?
   - Context – What are the significant background factors to this experience?
   - Clarify – What are the key processes (for reflection) in this experience?
2. Reflection:
   - What was I trying to achieve?
   - Why did I intervene as I did?
   - What were the consequences of my actions for:
     - myself
     - the patient/family
     - the people I work with?
   - How did I feel about this experience when it was happening?
   - How did the patient feel about it?
   - How do I know how the patient felt about it?
3. Influencing factors:
   - What internal factors influenced my decision-making?
   - What external factors influenced my decision-making?
   - What sources of knowledge did/should have influenced my decision-making?
4. Could I have dealt better with the situation?
   - What other choices did I have?
   - What would be the consequences of these other choices?
5. Learning:
   - How do I *now* feel about this experience?
   - How have I made sense of this experience in light of past experiences and future practice?
   - How has this experience challenged my ways of knowing:
     - empirics
     - aesthetics
     - ethics
     - personal?

as being a cycle, although it should really be seen as a spiral. Despite their structural differences, the Johns and Gibbs models are similar in character and have the same core components. These are:

- A description of events
- An evaluation of your feelings about the events
- An analysis of the events
- Thinking about future needs or developments.

> **Tip**
>
> Take some time to look at the two frameworks (Boxes 8.1, 8.2) and try writing the same event you wish to reflect upon with both to see which one you prefer.

When using a framework you should use the headings it provides and ask and answer the questions that are posed. You need to use all the steps identified in the framework in sequence in order to reflect upon an event.

Types of reflection

Schon (1999) identified two modes of reflection:

- 'Reflection in action' when the practitioner rethinks an immediate problem and alters or modifies their practice to solve it
- 'Reflecting on action' which is a more contemplative activity where issues are explored in depth after the event, out of which appropriate alterations are proposed for future events.

With reflection on action there is the benefit of distance from the event in terms of time and usually place, thus allowing a less obstructive or emotive view. However, although this 'after the event' mode of reflection might have advantages, there are times when practitioners must think about a situation and adjust their actions there and then.

Try to think of how you have reflected doing something that needed more or less instant solutions to a problematic situation and also when you have thought after an event on how you could do something differently in future. For example, reflection in action might occur when you are experiencing difficulties explaining a procedure to a patient and you realise that the patient needs you to draw diagrams to help them understand. When reflecting on action you might realise how important visual images are when communicating information to a patient, as it would be difficult for you to learn about human biology without diagrams or pictures. You might conclude that in future you should always be ready to draw diagrams to enhance your explanations.

Reflecting on difficult situations

When you look back on your time in a placement area some of your experiences may seem perplexing and, given the nature of health care, they might also be distressing. Coming face to face with harsh realities can be upsetting. As a student you may not feel ready to deal with events such as the death of a patient. Unfortunately, these things do occur as they are part of nursing and midwifery. On the other hand, there will be many things that you observe which you had not expected but with hindsight are clearly good learning experiences. Some things, although they might have seemed negative at the time, can be seen in a different light when thought through at a later date. However, you can sometimes help resolve your feelings and grow personally and professionally by the process of reflection.

> **Tip**
>
> Try to discuss distressing issues with someone experienced such as your mentor or personal tutor. They can provide the support you may need.

Using the first person when writing reflectively

It is common practice to write in the third person (i.e. not to use 'I') in academic essays (see p. 114). However, writing reflectively about professional practice is different in that it is acceptable to use the first person, although this does not mean you can write in a more colloquial style. You are writing about your experiences, and using 'I' will make the narrative more realistic. Trying to describe your feelings and emotions will sound stilted if you use 'the author' instead of 'I'.

> **Tip**
>
> Have a look at different types of articles in nursing journals – see when the authors use the first, second or third person.

If you wish to move your reflection to a discussion of theory it may be appropriate to switch between first and third person. This can be done in one piece of writing (Fairbairn & Winch 1996). It is like a presenter on television describing something in a detached tone, then turning to the audience and speaking directly with more intimate observations. Writing reflectively in the first person has a degree of intimacy in that it helps make the reader more attuned to your personal experience but this should not signal a change in tone to using slang or colloquial language.

Finally, although reflective accounts written as part of assignments can be in the first person, they do not have to include highly personal feelings. Always think carefully when disclosing your personal feelings about others as this may appear in a disingenuous light and consequently reflect badly on you as a professional. For example, you may personally disapprove of a person's lifestyle but, although you can acknowledge this, you should not be overly critical. These feelings can be kept in a personal reflective journal or diary and only appropriate extracts need be used in essays.

Keeping a reflective diary or journal

The terms diary and journal are often used interchangeably. A diary can be a daily record of planned events such as meetings or it can be a highly personal account of life events. The term journal can mean the same thing or it can be a professional magazine, e.g. *British Journal of Nursing*, which is commercially produced and contains research articles. Some people keep detailed accounts of their lives with the intention of publishing these at a later point, e.g. politicians, whereas others keep them for entirely personal purposes. The intention is that you can relive events at a later date and that they are not forgotten over time. Not everyone keeps a journal and you may feel it is too intrusive or just something you have never done before. The idea of writing down what you did may seem embarrassing and you may not have been used to writing in the first person. Keeping a diary or journal may be a new concept or something that you consider you would keep secret and personal.

If your journal is a personal initiative, there should usually be no reason why you would be asked to show it to anyone. You should regard it as a store of ideas and exact memories that you can return to at a later date to aid your learning. You might like to think of it as 'a learning log' and, as a record of your experiences as a student, it can be an effective learning tool. However, some courses may require you to submit your journal or learning log as part of an assessment. If this is the case you will be given guidelines as to what is expected.

If the feeling 'I hate the idea of keeping a journal' persists in your mind, you can try to overcome this by making an easy start. Try writing one or two short descriptive accounts of your experiences in placement per week. Once you get used to this, it should not be too painful and you can start to add phrases that identify gaps in your knowledge and your intentions to look up further information on a subject. Do not worry about how it looks; just think of it as a notebook of your thoughts. This will allow you to make a concrete start to reflection.

> **Tip**
>
> Remember there is nothing like practice: the more you write, the more confident you should feel about your writing capabilities.

Why keep a reflective journal?

A journal or reflective diary can be used to record experiences of professional practice and, as such, they are often recommended as a device to aid learning: 'Journal writing is extremely useful in recording professional development' (Bulman & Schutz 2004: 101).

According to Usher et al. (1999), although students often don't understand why they should keep a journal, there are a number of benefits if they do. Therefore it is important that we consider the benefits. Writing a journal will:

- Help your academic writing for assignments if you use it to practise
- Help you to reflect in a structured manner and improve the quality of your reflections (Jasper 1999)
- Identify issues that you don't understand and therefore focus your personal study
- Help you reflect upon your learning in practice by identifying areas for development
- Give you positive feedback when you identify areas where your practice was effective and appropriate.

What should be in a reflective journal?

A journal that is focused on your learning in the university and on placement can be a valuable source of material for assignments and your portfolio (see p. 180). Some areas you might like to include are:

- Your communications or interactions with patients, e.g. what you learned from talking to a patient about their illness or problems
- Nursing skills that you have observed or been taught to undertake, e.g. measuring blood pressures or giving injections
- Your ability to manage situations and provide handovers, e.g. how you helped a patient to have a wash in bed, or discussed at report the progress that a patient who you had been allocated to care for has made during a shift
- Investigations, procedures and treatments that you have observed, e.g. an X-ray or ultrasound
- Issues related to professional or ethical dilemmas, e.g. a patient who refuses to have a bath when you feel this care is needed.

> **Tip**
>
> Remember that the purpose of your reflective journal is to help you learn, not feel bad about things that you could have done differently. Try to be honest about areas where you feel you need to improve – but also give yourself credit when you do things well.

Descriptions of events in practice may provide you with areas that you need to link with theory. Alternatively, you may explore wider issues in your diary such as psychosocial, cultural or ethical factors, or political or economic aspects, all of which have an effect on nursing care.

Confidentiality

You must ensure that anyone mentioned in the journal, e.g. staff, other students, relatives and patients, is not identified or identifiable. The journal itself would normally be considered a private document (unless it is part of a course assessment) as there may be some items you do not wish to share. Nevertheless, do be careful of inappropriate expressions. Circumspection is essential, even if intended entirely for private consumption. As noted by Hull et al (2005), this is because there is always the possibility that incriminating information contained in a private journal/diary may be required by order of a court in a case of professional misconduct.

Malpractice

When writing about their experiences students occasionally realise that what they observed was poor professional practice. If you observe poor practice – such as a patient being mistreated, or you feel you have been mistreated in any way – you must talk to your mentor, the nurse in charge, your personal tutor or the link lecturer for the clinical area. It is important that you tell someone.

Tip

If you ever feel that you have witnessed neglect or professional misconduct it is important to report it to an appropriate person. It is never appropriate to inform the press, media or other bodies as this inevitably involves a breach of confidentiality. Your personal tutor or practice facilitator will make sure that the incident is properly investigated.

SUMMARY OF KEY POINTS

- Your portfolio is your record of your achievements as a student and this should be continued in your career as a registered nurse.
- Reflection is a tool that can be used to help us make sense of and learn from our experiences.
- Reflective frameworks can provide the basis for a systematic review of experiences.
- Developing your reflective skills through keeping a reflective journal is an essential part of learning effectively from the experience of nursing, both as a student and as a professional.

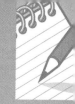

9

How to have confidence with numbers

Learning outcomes

This chapter will help you to learn how to:

- Check your numeracy skills and identify learning needs
- Understand the basics of working with numbers
- Develop your confidence with decimals, fractions and percentages
- Apply basic maths to calculate dosages of medicines.

INTRODUCTION

All areas of clinical practice require practitioners to be numerate. Numeracy means skill with numbers and embraces subjects within the discipline of mathematics such as arithmetic and geometry, as well as the ability to present and interpret numerical data. The level of numeracy required of a nurse varies from clinical area to clinical area but all nurses need to be able to work with numbers in order to calculate doses of medicines and other activities such as monitoring fluid balance. This chapter is aimed at those who want to develop their basic numeracy and provides examples and exercises that will help. If you feel confident about your numeracy abilities, you may just want to quickly review this chapter so that you get an idea of the skills you are likely to need as a nurse.

Numeracy is often regarded as a complex subject, with many people declaring themselves 'not very good at maths' and lacking in confidence. In addition, most of us use relatively little mathematics in our everyday lives and therefore our opportunity to improve is rather limited. It can come as a bit of a shock to the system when we are presented with unfamiliar problems that require maths to solve them. In fact, most of us do use maths in our everyday lives; we are just so used to doing it we don't realise. Take, for example, shopping for a new suit. If you see a suit in one shop for £250, and then the same suit in another shop for £230 most people would be able to identify that a) the suit in the second shop is cheaper and b) the difference in the price is £20.

Similarly, most people are aware that '50% off' means that something is half its normal price. The majority of people can add up their bank balances and know the difference between being in credit and being overdrawn. Likewise, if going on a journey of 120 miles with an average speed of 60 miles per hour, most drivers would be able to calculate that the journey will take 2 hours.

The type of maths described above is the same as that required in many clinical nursing situations. If you can cope with this maths, you probably have sufficient numeracy skills to function as a nurse.

Maths problems

Maths-based problems require us to have three distinct skills, i.e. the ability to:

- Perform the basic mathematical functions, e.g. to add and subtract
- Determine which mathematical functions (or processes) are required to solve the mathematical problem, i.e. realising when you need to divide or multiply
- Apply the numeracy skill in context, e.g. working out the exact dosage of a medicine.

Taking the example above of buying a new suit, the basic maths function you need to able to do is subtraction, the process that you need to be able to do is subtract the smaller value from the larger value and know that the resulting number is the difference in the two values, and the context in which this takes place is of course shopping. Now try the example shown in Box 9.1.

> ## Box 9.1 Example of mathematical functions
>
> Look at the example below; see if you can identify the different skills.
>
> Ram Patel is visiting his home in Oxford. He is travelling by bus from London. If the distance is 68 miles and the bus travels at an average speed of 51 miles per hour, how long will the journey take?

One of the issues we have in relation to these skills or stages is that we all take short-cuts, and our ability to show what we can do often depends on the situation and context of what we are doing. In other words, a nurse who can quite comfortably calculate the amount of substance to inject may not be able to solve the same equation when it is presented as a straightforward mathematical problem. This inability to perform maths in different situations is very common and tends to relate to how we identify the process(es) needed to achieve the desired outcome. In unfamiliar circumstances we may simply not recognise the shortcuts we normally take or be able to identify quite what we have to do.

Thus, when presented with a drugs calculation for the first time you will not be the only one thinking, 'I can't do that!' Instead you should think, 'I can do basic maths so this problem is within my ability but I need to practise to become familiar with the new situation I am working in.' However, one thing is sure: if you are not confident with the basic maths functions you will not be able to perform drug calculations correctly and are unlikely to understand basic health care information. This chapter is designed to help you get to grips with basic maths so that you can confidently tackle calculations in your career as a nurse.

Improving your basic maths skills

In everyday nursing, you will need to be able to do the following without the use of a calculator:

- Add
- Subtract
- Multiply
- Divide
- Understand decimals and decimal points
- Understand percentages
- Understand basic aspects of probability
- Understand how to calculate using simple fractions
- Convert between different units of measurement.

More advanced practice may require more maths skills, particularly if you undertake research that uses statistics. You might be wondering why you can't use a calculator. This is for two reasons: 1) because in practice a calculator may not always be available to you, and 2) because if you always use a calculator you do not develop a sense of what the correct answer should be. Therefore, if an error is made in calculating, you are less likely to spot it. Below we have outlined some ideas for improving your *basic* maths skills. Most people do have these basic skills, so don't panic.

Practise every day

At first, you will probably find that your maths skills are a little rusty so practice is important. Set yourself some sums; make sure you do any day-to-day maths tasks in your head. Try to give yourself small problems to solve as they occur daily in your life. For example, when you go shopping, try calculating the amount of change you are due before it is shown on the till. If you shop at a supermarket, add up the bill as you go along and see how close you are to the answer. If you have children and pay each term for school meals, calculate how much the bill is per week and then per meal. Regularly doing this sort of activity will help you develop and sharpen your skills. Straker (1995–1996) has produced a series of books called *Mental Maths*; using these books will help you to develop your abilities to perform numerical skills without needing a calculator or pen and paper. If you are unsure of your abilities and want to test your skills, the website www.mathcentre.ac.uk contains excellent tutorial material and suitable quick tests; www.move-on.org.uk gives you access to both informal and formal test systems.

If you find it difficult to give yourself challenges, try buying a basic school revision guide; you probably need to buy one aimed at older schoolchildren (e.g. *Practice in the Basic Skills: Maths*, a series by Newton & Smith 2003). There are also some books aimed at adult learners (e.g. Lawler 2003). In addition, there are many useful maths tutorial websites such as www.bbc.co.uk/schools/ks3bitesize/maths and www.bbc.co.uk/schools/11_16/maths.shtml.

You may also find some of the CD-ROMs on the market worth exploring. The presentation may seem patronising, but they are useful and sitting down at a computer to work on a CD-ROM does give you dedicated practice time.

Learning by heart

Sometimes learning answers by heart helps us to solve mathematical problems and can also help some people to get a better feel for numbers. It's a good idea to know your multiplication tables (up to 10 times table) by heart, and knowing the product of pairs of numbers from 1 to 20 can enhance your ability to add and subtract. For example, $7 + 8 = 15$; $14 + 14 = 28$; $15 + 17 = 32$; $3 + 12 = 15$; $7 + 19 = 26$, and so on.

The number line

One way to think about numbers is to imagine that they are strung out on a line with each number being an equal distance from the next. The line starts at 0 and carries on forever:

$$0\ 1\ 2\ 3\ 4\ 5\ 6\ 7\ 8\ 9\ 10\ 11\ 12\ 13\ 14\ 15\ 16\ 17\ 18\ 19\ 20 \ldots$$

From this number line, we can visualise calculations. We can see, for example, that 3 is the number that is three units of distance from 0, and if we move on three more units we come to the number 6. Thus we can see that $3 + 3 = 6$. We can also see that 2×3 is the same result as moving two units three times – the answer, of course, is 6 units of distance. Similarly, if we are asked to divide 6 by 2, we are being asked to say how many times two units of distance would fit into six units of distance – the answer is 3. Visualising problems in this way can really help you get to grips with the basics and develop the confidence to tackle problems that are more complex.

When we write numbers using the decimal system (base 10), we record the number of units – 10s, 100s, 1000s, etc. – in the number. So 328 really means 3 hundreds, 2 tens and 8 units (Fig. 9.1). You need to make sure you are familiar with this system of numbers. It is particularly important when considering calculations that involve values that are not whole numbers.

Multiplication

As we said in the previous section, to know your multiplication tables by heart is very helpful. If the multiplication is complex, write it down and use a method you have confidence in. Let's look at the calculation 8×36, outlined in Box 9.2.

Box 9.2

Step 1: Write out the calculation

$$\frac{38}{6} \times$$

Step 2: Multiply the units on the top line (first number from the right) by the units on the bottom line

$8 \times 6 = 48$

Step 3: You can now put the units from this calculation (8) into the space for the answer and you will need to carry 4 tens. We cannot place these tens onto the result line yet, because so far we are only working with the units, and there may be more tens to deal with. To remind yourself of the tens you are carrying, write them as a subscript adjacent to the units

$$\frac{38}{4^6} \times$$
$$8$$

Step 4: Multiply the tens on the top line by the units on the bottom line

$6 \times 3 = 18$. Remember that what you are doing here is in fact multiplying 6×30; this is because the second column represents tens

Step 5: We must now add any tens we were carrying to the 18 we have just calculated

In total then we have $18 + 4$ tens. This equals 22

Step 6: Add the total number of tens to the overall answer

$$\frac{38}{6} \times$$
$$\overline{228}$$

If this were a multiplication of larger numbers we would use the process outlined on page 201. But before we look at multiplying larger numbers, here are a few tricks to help with multiplying, however large or small the numbers are.

Doubling and halving

One trick for any multiplication calculation is to try what is called 'doubling and halving'. The idea behind this is to try to manipulate the sum so that the numbers are a little easier to handle. To double and half you double one of the numbers and half the other; it doesn't matter which as long as you remember that, whatever you do to one number, you do the opposite to the other. For example, if you were doing the calculation 38 × 8, we could change this by 'doubling and halving' to 76 × 4, or 18 × 16. To us 76 × 4 looks a much easier calculation than 18 × 16. The beauty of 'doubling and halving' is you can continue it until you get to the answer. Thus from 76 × 4, just double 76 and halve 4; this gives 152 × 2, and doing the 'doubling and halving' again gives 304 × 1, which is, of course, the answer. 'Doubling and halving' becomes more useful and easier as you become more familiar with numbers.

Estimating the answer

Calculators are often used in the clinical setting but how will you know if the calculator has given the correct answer (calculators seldom get the answer wrong; it will be much more likely that you have hit the wrong button on the calculator). In order to check you will need some idea of the answer and this can be gained through estimation. If dealing with a calculation such as 8 × 38, one method of estimation is to alter the numbers slightly to numbers that are easy to deal with. For example, if we mentally nudge the 8 up to 10, all we then need to do is the mental calculation 10 times 38, which is easier because, when multiplying by 10, all you need to do is add a 0 to the number being multiplied. Thus, the estimation is that the value should be in the region of 380. Now you might think that this is quite a long way off the correct answer, but the estimation is there as a safety device to reduce risk; it gives an idea of the type of value that should be anticipated. Without an estimation there would be a risk of making a serious clinical error, e.g. if the calculator had said 3040. When you estimate, it is always a good idea to round up or down to numbers with which you feel more confident.

Multiplying larger numbers

Let's look at a harder calculation this time: 75 × 28 (Box 9.3). We follow the same process as in the first calculation although this time we add extra steps because we are multiplying by a value that has both units and tens.

Notice how the use of this 'long multiplication' method means that, at each step, the maths is simple; you just need to know your times table and a bit of addition.

Let's look again at the shortcuts that we could use. We could double and halve, so instead of 75 × 28 we have 150 × 14; doubling and halving again would give

Box 9.3

Step 1: Write out the calculation

$$\frac{75}{28} \times$$

Step 2: Multiply the units in the top line by the units on the bottom line (8 × 5). Put any units into the space for the answer. Because 8 × 5 gives 40, 0 is entered into the units; 4 tens are carried over

$$\frac{75}{2_48} \times$$
$$0$$

Step 3: Just as before now multiply the lower units by the upper tens (8 × 7). Note that 8 × 7 gives 56 but we carried 4 tens from before: hence 600

There is a general rule to be seen here: when doing long multiplication always multiply out the whole of the top line by the units before moving on to the tens

$$\frac{75}{28} \times$$
$$600$$

Step 4a: Now repeat, only this time, for the tens. The result goes on the line beneath that for the units and, when we start, we add a zero into the first column of the new results row

$$\frac{75}{28} \times$$
$$600$$
$$0$$

Step 4b: First multiply the units (2 × 5) and add to the new result line

$$\frac{75}{_128} \times$$
$$600$$
$$00$$

Because the answer was 10 we add a zero to the tens column and carry over 100

Step 5: Multiply the tens in the lower row by the tens in the upper row (i.e. 2 × 7) and then add the result to the new results row (do not forget any 100s now being carried)

$$\frac{75}{28} \times$$
$$600$$
$$1500$$

Step 6: The last step is to add the two lines of the results together

$$2100$$

300 × 7. Multiplying 300 × 7 is relatively straightforward because we can use a shortcut. The only digits involved are 3 and 7 and if you know your 7 times table you will know that 7 × 3 = 21. You need to remember, however, that you are multiplying by 300, not just by 3, so you add all the zeros to the end of your multiplication – hence the answer of 2100. You can use this trick whenever you are dealing with numbers that are multiples of 10, 100, 1000, etc. Look at the sum 100 × 200: all we need do is 2 × 1 = 2 then add the zeros back on so the answer is 20,000.

Introduction

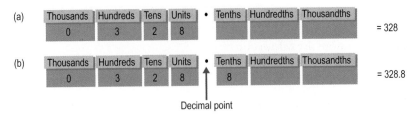

	Thousands	Hundreds	Tens	Units	•	Tenths	Hundredths	Thousandths	
(a)	0	3	2	8					= 328

	Thousands	Hundreds	Tens	Units	•	Tenths	Hundredths	Thousandths	
(b)	0	3	2	8		8			= 328.8

Decimal point

Figure 9.1 The decimal system

Multiplying decimals and fractions

At some point in your nursing career you will almost certainly have to multiply something by a fraction or work with decimal points, e.g. when calculating drug dosages per unit of body weight. Most of your work with fractions will be quite simple but if you want to use your calculator you will need to be able to convert fractions to decimals because calculators cannot work with fractions (see p. 205).

A decimal strictly means one-tenth and decimal numbers are those that are not whole numbers (integers) but are numbers that are made up of part of whole numbers. Thus 328.5 would be a decimal made up of 3 hundreds 2 tens 8 units and 5 tenths (see Fig. 9.1b). One whole unit is made up of 10 tenths, just as 100 is made up of 10 tens.

Great care is required when working with decimals as misplacing the decimal point can cause serious errors. It can produce a result that is multiples of 10 more or less than required. When using decimals, follow the normal pattern for multiplication and you shouldn't go wrong. Thus 75 × 2.9 would be written as shown in Box 9.4, care being taken to keep all the units, tens, hundreds, etc. in the appropriate columns. Box 9.4 demonstrates how to perform this calculation safely.

Now that you have the answer, stop and ask yourself if this result sounds about right. To do this you need to do an estimate (see p. 200). In this calculation you may notice that 2.9 is very close to the number 3, so you will be able to quickly work out that 3 × 75 is 225. The answer expected from multiplying 2.9 and 75 should therefore be slightly less than 225 (because 2.9 is slightly less than 3). Making estimates of the results of calculations is an important clinical skill. You should always try to estimate before you calculate; unexpected results can then be questioned.

Division

Division seems cause more problems than multiplication. This is strange because division is the mathematical opposite of multiplication. Division is asking the question, 'How many times do I need to multiply x to get to y?' If you think of a multiplication example, e.g. 3 × 6 = 18, this can be rearranged to give 3 = 18 divided by 6, or 18 divided by 3 = 6. Thus all multiplication and division is linked. This is an important relationship to remember as it occurs in many calculations.

The symbol most commonly used to denote the need for division is a forward slash (/), although a variety of methods can be used to set out the actual calculations. In nursing you will need to use division when calculating drug dosages, body mass index (BMI) and fluid balances.

Box 9.4

Step 1: Write out the calculation

$$\frac{75}{2.9} \times$$

Step 2: Multiply the smallest value numbers on the bottom line with the smallest on the top. In this example that is 9 × 5, which equals 45. But of course, this is really 4 units and 5 tenths. The 5 tenths are entered in the appropriate column in the line for the results and the 4 units are carried

$$\frac{75}{2_4.9} \times$$
$$.5$$

Step 3: Multiply the smallest units on the bottom line with the tens column on the next; the calculation is 9 × 7, giving us 63. We start to enter the 3 on the units line, but must remember we are carrying 4 units from Step 1, thus we enter 67, not 63

$$\frac{75}{2_4.9} \times$$
$$67.9$$

Step 4: We then repeat with the units

$$\frac{75}{2.9} \times$$
$$67.5$$
$$150.0$$

Notice how we recorded the latest calculation as 150.0 rather than just 150; this is simply to make sure that the columns stay in place, look neat and that the decimal point doesn't accidentally end up where it shouldn't

Step 5: The last step is to add the two lines of the results together

217.5

With a division such as 56/7, there are a number of ways to approach this. The simplest is to try to link it to your multiplication table; how many times 7 equals 56? The answer is 8. If you struggle with this initially, try using the 'subtraction method'. First write down the number 56 and subtract 7, repeat this until you reach 0, then simply count the number of times you subtracted 7. If your value does not divide exactly by the value you are dividing it by, you will end up producing a decimal (see p. 202).

Long division

Long division is simply the name given to division calculations that involve large numbers; it is called long division because the calculations tended to extend a long way down the page. The method we will describe is designed to save space. The example will use the calculation 374/11. When doing division by hand the calculation is normally set out as shown in Box 9.5.

Box 9.5

Step 1: Write out the calculation

$11\overline{)374}$

Step 2: Divide the first digit of the value being divided by the value you are dividing by (11 into 3); carry forward any numbers that cannot be divided to produce a whole number. In this example 3 is carried

$11\overline{)3^374}$

Step 3: Values carried forward are placed in front of the next digit and the resulting number is then divided by the value you are dividing by (in this example 11 into 37)

$11\overline{)3^37^44}$ ^3

Step 4 Place the 3 on the top of the equation. There are, however, 4 left over (37 – 33)

Step 5: Repeat the process, carrying the 4

$11\overline{)3^37^44}$ ^{34}

As 11 goes exactly into 44, the calculation is complete: the answer is 34

The example in Box 9.5 is a shorter version of long division as not all the stages are shown; you will notice that it assumes that the subtractions (to calculate how much is carried forward) are performed in your head. In the longer version, the subtractions are shown in full and the calculation goes down the page (Box 9.6).

Sometimes when doing division the value we obtain does not divide into the number exactly, in which case the answer will be a decimal, as shown in the calculation 58 divided by 7 (58/7) in Box 9.7. Of course, you will not always be able to tell whether a decimal will be produced before you start the calculation, but as soon as you begin to think that a decimal will be produced, using long division is wise. As with multiplication, when dealing with such calculations take care with how you write the values.

Unfortunately, for many divisions, there is no absolute solution, and you could carry on doing the division forever. Hence, at some point we stop and round up the result. Indeed, even when there is a solution, if this involves many values after the decimal point then we usually do not write down (express) all the values after the decimal point; it is conventional to write the answer to two or three decimal places (i.e. 8.28 or 8.286). The final digit should be rounded up or down according to the digit that follows. If the following digit is 5 or above it should be rounded up to the next whole number; if the following digit is below 5 it should be rounded down to the next whole number. In the example in Box 9.7 the complete calculation would be 8.28571429. To round it to three decimal places the 5 is increased to 6 because the following digit is greater than 5. Had the next digit been smaller than 5 the figure would have been rounded down to 8.284.

To know how many values to express you need to think about the accuracy of what you are measuring. For example, if you have taken six measurements of urine output over a period of time and you wish to express the average, you would only express the value in accordance with our original level of accuracy. So, if your

---

Box 9.6

Step 1: Write out the calculation%

$$11\overline{)374}$$

Step 2: Divide the first digit of the value being divided by the value you are dividing by (11 into 3). If this cannot be done, divide instead the value formed by the first two digits (in this case 37)

Step 3: Place the result (3) on top of the equation over the 7. Place the total amount that you divided 37 by, i.e. 33 (3×11) beneath the 37

$$\begin{array}{r} 3 \\ 11\overline{)374} \\ 33 \end{array}$$

Step 4: Subtract the 33 from the 37 to get the remainder, which is 4

$$\begin{array}{r} 3 \\ 11\overline{)374} \\ 33 \\ 4 \end{array}$$

Step 5: Bring down the digit not being used from the top line (4) and write it on the end of the remainder

$$\begin{array}{r} 3 \\ 11\overline{)374} \\ 33 \\ 44 \end{array}$$

Step 6: Divide 44 by 11 and place the value (4) on the result line next to the original 3

$$\begin{array}{r} 34 \\ 11\overline{)374} \\ 33 \\ 44 \end{array}$$

As 11 goes exactly into 44, the calculation is complete: the answer is 34

---

original results were expressed as millilitres it is unlikely that your measurement accuracy will ever be higher than 0.5 ml.

Fractions, decimals, percentages, ratios, proportions and probability

You may think it rather unusual to include so many different terms in one subsection; however, the point we are trying to make is that all these terms are linked and, to a large extent, can be and are used interchangeably. The first two (fractions and decimals) will be used in drug calculations, whereas the last four are often used in the reporting of the phenomena of illness and in the management of health services, e.g. the percentage of patients suffering from various conditions, chances of surviving, the proportions of the community from different ethnic groups, etc. Occasionally the concentration of a solution may also be expressed as a percentage.

Fractions

A fraction is simply one number divided by another. Most of the fractions we are used to dealing with (1/2, 1/4) tend to be numbers that are less than one. The number above the line is called the numerator and the number below the line is called the denominator. Fractions are involved in many calculations although we do not often recognise them as such. It is a good idea to try to understand some of the basics.

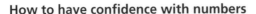

> **Box 9.7**
>
> **Step 1**: Write out the calculation
>
> $$7\overline{)58}$$
>
> **Step 2**: Divide the first digit of the value being divided by the value you are dividing by (7 into 5); carry forward any numbers that cannot be divided to produce a whole number. In this example 5 is carried
>
> $$7\overline{)5^58}$$
>
> **Step 3**: Values carried forward are placed in front of the next digit and the resulting number is then divided by the value you are dividing by (in this example 7 into 58)
>
> $$\frac{8}{7\overline{)5^58}}$$
>
> **Step 4**: Place the result (8) on the top of the equation. There are, however, 2 left over (58 – 56)
>
> $$\frac{8}{7\overline{)5^58^2}}$$
>
> There are now no new values to use. To get round this problem, place a decimal point on the top line and add a zero on the bottom line where the tenths should go. Add the decimal point to both the top and bottom rows
>
> **Step 5**: You can now repeat step 3 and divide 7 into 20; place the result on the top line
>
> $$\frac{8.}{7\overline{)5^58.^20}}$$
>
> **Step 6**: 7 goes into 20 two times and we have 6 left over (20 – 14). So 2 is placed on the result line and we repeat the process from Step 4
>
> $$\frac{8.2}{7\overline{)5^58.^20^60}}$$
>
> **Step 7**: Repeat until a solution is found
>
> For this division there is no absolute solution
>
> $$\frac{8.28}{7\overline{)5^58.^20^60^40}}$$

If we divide 1 by 8 we will get the answer 0.125 (a decimal). Fractions often have equivalents, i.e. they are written differently but when expressed as a decimal have the same value; for example, 30/60, 17/34, 12/24 and 1/2 when expressed as a decimal all have the same value, i.e. 0.5. Similarly, 3/9, 1/3, 6/18 and 9/27 can be expressed as 0.33.

To add fractions we must find a common number to link them. For example, to add 1/2 and 1/3 we must change them so that they have a common denominator (the same number on the bottom). In this case it would be 6. 1/2 expressed with a denominator of 6 becomes 3/6, and 1/3 becomes 2/6. Now the fractions can be added, because both are expressed with the same denominator. The answer is, of course, 5/6.

When multiplying fractions we simply multiply the numerators by each other then do the same with the denominator. For example:

$$\frac{6}{7} \times \frac{3}{5} = \frac{6 \times 3}{7 \times 5} = \frac{18}{35}$$

Fractions should be expressed in their simplest form, but it is not possible to reduce this fraction any further as there are no numbers that will divide exactly into 18 and into 35.

Dividing fractions

Dividing fractions is slightly more complex. What you do is invert the second fraction and then multiply the fractions together. For example:

To divide $\frac{6}{7} \div \frac{3}{5}$ invert the second fraction so that it becomes 5 over 3 and then multiply, i.e. $\frac{6 \times 5}{7 \times 3} = \frac{30}{21}$.

Notice in this case the resulting new fraction is larger than 1, i.e. 21 will go into 30 and there will be 9 left over. Fractions should be expressed in their most simple form. The result here could initially be expressed as 1 and 9/21. The fraction 9/21 can be simplified further by dividing by 3. Thus the result becomes 1 and 3/7 or 1⅗.

Proportions

Proportion refers to the amount of something in relation to the total amount of that factor, e.g. the proportion of women who visited their general practitioner (GP) in relation to the total number of people who visited. This proportion could be expressed as a fraction (e.g. 2/3 of the patients who visited the sexual health clinic were women) or in actual values (e.g. 21 clients visited the clinic today, 14 of whom were women).

If asked the question, 'What proportion of your time do you spend studying?' you are being asked to express how much time in relation to the whole. You would probably answer by using a fraction (e.g. 1/4) or perhaps a percentage (25%).

Percentages

A percentage is a number expressed as a part of or proportion of 100, i.e. whatever the total number of 'things' involved, we mathematically convert the total to equal 100. Per cent (%) actually means per 100, so 50 per cent is really 50/100; 50/100 is the same as 1/2, which is also the same as the decimal 0.5. Percentages are widely used and it is worthwhile spending time becoming accustomed to using them. You will find percentages used for many types of data ranging from the concentration of solutions, to the occurrence of certain types of disease, to the chance of dying from a particular condition or trauma.

To calculate a percentage all you need to do is express the proportion you are dealing with as a decimal and multiply the answer by 100. For example, if discussing chickenpox with a group of parents, you know that the incidence of the disease is about 1 in 32 of the population of 5 to 7-year-old children in any year. You may consider, however, that the parents are much more likely to be able to understand this information if it is given as a percentage. To calculate the percentage, first express 1/32 as a decimal, then multiply the answer by 100:

$$1/32 = 0.0312'5 \times 100 = 3.125.$$

Therefore, we can say that approximately 3.1% of 5 to 7-year-old children will get chickenpox in any year. The way that we express this type of information is very important to avoid unintentionally misleading.

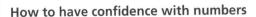

Think about how the security of contraceptive devices is described. We talk about devices as being 99.9% secure, which really means that, of 1000 women who use this method of contraception during the year, just one pregnancy is likely to occur. A contraceptive device called Persona® has been marketed as having a security level of 94%, or 6 unwanted pregnancies per 100 women using the device. This translates to a ratio of 1 unwanted pregnancy per 17 users per year. The message here is that the same values may seem different depending on how they are expressed; health professionals need to be familiar with these types of numbers and data.

Ratio

The last section raised two new concepts: ratio and probability. A ratio is a comparison of the amount of one phenomenon in relation to the amount of another. For example, the ratio of men to women is about 1:1, which means that for every man there is approximately one woman. Notice how this differs from a proportion, which in this example would be expressed as '50% of people are men'. From the scenario described earlier, if we were to express the difference in visits to the GP as a ratio we would say, 'The ratio of male to female clients was 1:2', i.e. for every one male client there are two female clients.

Probability

Probability is related to risk, a very important issue in health care. Probability is a measure of chance or risk. We quite often talk of probability in terms of percentages; for example, there is a 10% chance of an inpatient of an acute hospital getting a hospital-acquired infection (HAI). Sometimes this is expressed as a fraction, such as 1 in every 10 patients gets an HAI. Strictly speaking, however, probability should be expressed as a decimal between 0.0 and 1.0. If the probability of something is 0 it means it will never happen (the probability of winning the lottery if you don't buy a ticket) whereas if the probability is 1.0 it means it is certain to happen. Thus for our example based on HAIs, we could say the probability is 0.1. If you convert the decimal 0.1 to a percentage (see p. 207) the answer will be 10%.

Units of measurement (SI units)

The units of measurement used in health care are standard units called SI units, e.g. metres and kilograms. SI stands for *Système International d'unités*, an internationally recognised system for units of measurement. Each unit of measurement has a central unit (its SI unit): for linear measures we use the metre; for weight we use the kilogram. Sometimes SI units are not easy to use because they are too big (we would not refer to amounts of medicine in terms of kilograms) or too small. SI units have multiples or subunits, some of which you will find familiar, e.g. kilometres are a multiple of metres and centimetres are a subunit of metres. Similarly, grams and milligrams are subdivisions of the kilogram. The various multiples and subdivisions of SI units use standard prefixes, e.g. kilo. A prefix is a group of letters that is added to the beginning of a word to change its meaning.

Each prefix denotes how many times the unit is smaller or larger than the unit denoted in the suffix (in this case the suffix is the part of the word that normally

Table 9.1 SI units commonly used in health care

Prefix	What it does to suffix	Symbol
Kilo	×1000	k
Deci	÷10	d
Centi	÷100	c
Milli	÷1000	m
Micro	÷100,000	μ
Nano	÷100,000,000	n

designates the SI unit). Thus, kilogram has the prefix 'kilo' and the suffix 'gram'. Because kilo means 'multiply by 1000' a kilogram is 1000 times larger than a gram. All SI units use the same prefixes and the same symbol to denote that prefix. You need to remember those most commonly used (Table 9.1). However, some commonly used units are not strictly speaking SI units – a good example is the litre – although the same applies for the naming of this unit and its subunits.

When using weight the common units used are in multiples of 1000. So a milligram (mg) is 1000th of a gram and a microgram (mcg) is 1000th of a milligram. This fact is useful to remember when converting between different units of measurement.

Converting from smaller to larger units

To convert from a smaller to a larger unit you must *divide* the smaller unit by the magnitude of the difference between the units. If converting milligrams to grams, you divide the amount in milligrams by 1000. Thus 2000 mg is the same as 2 g.

Converting from larger to smaller units

Similarly, when converting a larger unit to a smaller unit you must *multiply* by the magnitude of the difference between the units. If converting grams to milligrams you multiply by 1000. Thus 1.5 g would become 1500 mg.

Tip

Be careful when using abbreviations for units of measurement. In general, micrograms and nanograms should be written out in full. If you are ever in doubt about what has been written, you must ask.

Checking your numeracy skills

Having worked through this chapter you should now have a good idea of your level of skill and any learning needs. Which of the statements in Box 9.8 best sums up/matches how you feel about your numeracy skills?

Box 9.8

I can perform calculations with my calculator, and I get them right. I tend to get a little confused when I have to do calculations in my head

This means ... Your fundamental numeracy skills are good, but you have low levels of confidence and mental arithmetic skills. Given that you clearly understand what you should do to get the correct answers you need to improve your mental arithmetic skills. Start by doing calculations on paper and write out each step. Your mental arithmetic skills will improve with practice. After a while you will need paper less and less, but when doing important calculations write out the answers step by step.

I thought I was OK at maths; I've worked in a shop and had to help customers work out how much material they needed to buy. I just go a bit blank when people mention drug calculations. I just don't get it

This means ... Your fundamental skills are good; your issue seems to be transferring skills from one context to another. You may struggle to apply your abilities until you can see and do calculations in practice. You need to practise your calculation skills in more realistic circumstances. Take opportunities to do calculations in practice and use any simulations available to you.

I'm really panicking now; I can't get the right answers even when I use my calculator. I have never been any good at maths

This means ... You are right to be concerned; it is good that you have identified this issue. It would seem that you have problems with your fundamental numeracy skills. You need to seek advice from your personal tutor or learning support unit. Look at some of the self-help guides suggested in this book. Give yourself time to practise your maths: focus first on fundamentals, (multiplication, etc.) and then later set yourself realistic practice calculations. It may help to observe calculations being undertaken and used in practice so that you get a good idea of what is required.

Using numeracy skills in nursing practice

This book primarily concerns study skills rather than performing calculations but we recognise that students sometimes find drug calculations a little intimidating. Therefore, in the following section, we outline some of the basic calculations and issues that you are likely to come across when administering medicine. This will allow you to put into practice some of the maths functions that have been described earlier in this chapter. Further information about calculating drug doses and intravenous (IV) infusion rates can be found in Nicol et al (2004).

The most common errors that nurses make in practice are to do with sorting out what maths actually needs to be carried out. As Arnold (1998) found, nurses can do the maths required but have problems deciding what processes (e.g. whether to divide or multiply) are required. This issue is sometimes called conceptualisation: put more simply, setting out the problem. As stated earlier, forming the problem to be solved is the critical step.

The aim of the drug administration process is to ensure that the patient receives the amount and form of a drug that has been prescribed, at the appropriate time and in appropriate circumstances (e.g. with food). The calculation 'problem' concerns ensuring that the amount administered is correct. On the surface the issue is very simple; however, the problem arises when the size of tablet or the concentration of solution does not match up with that prescribed.

The outline of the problem is, 'How much/many of the particular available unit of the drug do I need in order to administer the amount prescribed?' The next step is to form that problem so that it can be solved. We now need to express this problem in a way in which we can apply real values and numbers.

Calculating the number of tablets or capsules required

In order to determine how many units are needed in order to administer the prescribed amount of drug, we need to know the number of units required. We already know (from the prescription) the amount in the unit. To answer this question we are interested in how many of one thing fits into another, i.e. how many units of the drug are needed to fit the prescription. When we ask 'how many' of anything it means that we need to divide what we want to administer by the amount in the unit available. If, for example, the prescription states two tablets and the unit available is a single tablet, then it is easy to see that the answer is 2 divided by 1 which equals two tablets.

When administering medicine, the amount you want is the prescribed amount, what you have is the unit the medicine comes in and what you need to know is the number of those units. The following equation is used to sum this up:

$$\frac{\text{amount prescribed (what you want)}}{\text{amount in the unit}} = \text{number required}$$

In practice, the prescription will usually be written as a dose (e.g. 10 mg) and the strength of each tablet will be known. Thus, if you are asked to administer 1000 mg of paracetamol and you had 500 mg tablets, the equation would be:

$$2 = \frac{1000\,\text{mg}}{500\,\text{mg}}$$

The process outlined is common to most of the drug calculations you will need to perform. We do not recommend that you try to remember the equation but do try to focus on the basic principle, i.e. if you want to know how many of something you need to fit into something else, you are talking about dividing what you want by the amount in the unit you have. This principle applies when you are trying to calculate how many tablets you need. For more information on drug calculations, see Lapham and Agar (2003); for IV calculations, see Nicol et al (2004).

Breaking tablets

Occasionally you will find that the amount prescribed is less than that of the unit available, in which case the tablet needs to be split. In general, you can only do

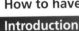

this when the tablet is scored, i.e. has a line across designed to enable it to be broken cleanly into two. If you are not sure that it will divide evenly you should consult a pharmacist and check the prescription.

> **Tip**
>
> Always double check that the result of your calculation is reasonable. If the answer to your calculation suggests that you need to administer 20 tablets, you have probably done the calculation incorrectly – it is very unlikely that anyone would prescribe more than two tablets. If your answer does not make sense, ask someone to check your calculation. Unusual answers must be treated with caution because they are probably wrong; you must request clarification from a senior colleague or the prescriber.

Converting units to aid calculation

You may find that that an amount prescribed is in different units from the amount available in the tablet or capsule. In the above example the prescription could have said 1 g rather than 1000 mg. Thus, you need to be able to convert between units (see p. 209). When calculating, convert all the values in the equation into the same units before performing the calculations. In general, convert values into the smallest unit being used (otherwise you will find yourself needing to use decimals). If you are asked to administer 1 gram of a substance that is only available in 500 mg tablets, convert all the values to milligrams (mg) before performing the calculations.

SUMMARY OF KEY POINTS

- Most people use maths in their everyday lives and practising every day (e.g. working out in your head how much change you should receive) will develop your skill.
- Knowing your multiplication tables really helps with mental arithmetic.
- It is important to estimate the answer in your head, even if using a calculator, as this will alert you if you make a calculation error.
- In nursing, you need to be able to do straightforward maths in your head, e.g. when calculating how many tablets are required.
- Write your calculations out in full so you can check that each step is correct.
- An understanding of percentages, proportions, probability and ratio is helpful when interpreting health information and reading research studies.
- Understanding the prefixes (e.g. kilo, micro) when using SI units can help you when converting them to larger or smaller units.

Glossary

This glossary has been designed to help you to quickly grasp the meaning of words used in this book and those that you may come across early in your career as a nurse.

Academic registrar: this person has overall responsibility for ensuring that all the procedures related to programme results are correctly recorded and that qualifications awarded meet the standards.

Academic style: a mode of writing that is formal, uses precise terms, is impersonal and usually, though not exclusively, written in the third person.

Access course: a UK-based programme of study to allow those who do not have standard entrance qualifications to enter the nursing profession.

Affective learning: learning that helps students to value the phenomena about which they are learning.

Analysis: the activity of breaking down an issue or an argument into its component parts. Analysis is a term often used in relation to learning outcomes and written assignments.

Andragogy: the study of how adults learn.

APEL: Accreditation of Prior Experiential Learning. This is a formal assessment of learning from experiences. Such learning can often be credited towards achieving a qualification.

Assessment: a process used to determine the level and amount of learning that has occurred.

Assessor: a person who measures a performance against criteria and makes a judgement in relation to competence.

Assignment: this is a task to be completed and may be used interchangeably with the term assessment.

Bibliography: a written list of sources of information used by an author when preparing a text; can also be a list of useful publications.

Cognitive skills: a general term for skills that require mental agility, e.g. solving problems.

Competence: the ability to safely and adeptly perform a skill to a required standard.

Competencies: set standards, often nationally agreed, which demand a performance using knowledge and skills.

Concept: an idea or notion, often with universal acceptance (e.g. accountability with health professions).

Confidentiality: keeping information about a patient secure for use within the care team (never identify patients when completing assessments).

Continuing professional development: education and training activities that are carried out after a professional qualification has been obtained. It includes activities such as formally organised courses and self-directed study.

Credit (academic): used in higher education to designate the amount and level of learning that has taken place during a period (e.g. module) of study.

Critical analysis: the process of looking at aspects of an argument, issue or action to determine if the constituent parts are true and conclusions or reasoning valid.

Critique: the process of examining the issues surrounding a phenomenon to determine if the supporting reasoning and explanations are valid.

Curricula (or curriculum): the areas of study that make up a course or pro-gramme of study.

Deferred: this term may refer to an assignment result that is neither a pass nor a final fail result, as the student is given an opportunity to resubmit an improved version of the assignment for another attempt.

Describe: to give an objective account of the known detail of a process, procedure, object, emotion, event or concept.

Discuss: a term used often in learning outcomes and assessments. Normally means to examine in detail, giving different views and arguments concerning a particular issue.

Dissertation: extensive written coursework that is usually research based and completed as part of a degree course.

Download: a term used to describe transferring information (files, pictures, music) from one computer system (e.g. internet) to another (e.g. your own).

E Learning: a method of learning/study that is organised and delivered using com-puter technology.

Essay: a detailed, structured, written account of a subject, phenomenon or issue.

Explain: give the reasons behind a phenomenon, process or procedure.

Extension: this term is often used in adult education to mean allowing extra time for an assignment (e.g. an essay) to be completed. Most universities have policies with regard to granting extensions.

Facilitator: a person who assists students to learn in a manner that encourages learning. This is more developmental than directly teaching a student (*see also* Mentor).

Feedback: comments made on performance, designed to help you develop your abilities; can be given orally or in writing.

Formative assignment: a method of assessing progress where the grade and marker's comments are intended to provide feedback. The marks given do not count towards a formal pass grade or degree.

Goals: a statement of expected or intended achievement.

Grammar and syntax: the structure and order of sentences.

Guidelines: an indication of the processes or procedures that should be followed.

Index: a device that indicates where items (e.g. in a book) can be found.

Induction: in relation to the workplace or placements this is a process of introduction to a role or environment. Induction usually includes making you aware of relevant polices and procedures.

Journal (diary): an alternative word for a diary, e.g. a reflective journal.

Journal (publication): printed collection of articles on a scientific or technical subject, usually containing research published at regular intervals, e.g. monthly.

Learning aims: a broad statement of the learning to be achieved during a period of study.

Learning contract: a written agreement between a learner and mentor/tutor, which specifies the learning outcomes for a period of time and the actions that will be taken by both parties to achieve these outcomes.

Learning outcome or objectives: a precise statement of the expected acquired learning following a period of instruction (*see also* Goals, Learning aims).

Lecture: a formal, verbal presentation of a subject by an expert. There is usually no dialogue between the lecturer and the audience although some questions may be asked at the end of the talk.

Legislation: law passed by parliament. This may be national (e.g. Nurses and Midwives Act 1992) or international (e.g. European Union (EU) Manual Handling Regulations 1993).

Literate: ability to read and write, often expressed as 'level of literacy'.

Literature review: a process of finding and critically analysing the published information concerning a topic.

Mentor: one who supports, guides and advises. Mentors can be formally named persons or, in the more general meaning of the word, you may select someone to act as an informal mentor. When on clinical placement you will have a named mentor who is normally allocated to you by the area manager.

Mitigating or extenuating circumstances: general terms given to reasons that may lead to poorer than predicted performance on an assessment.

Module: an organised period of study with a specific title, content and assessment(s). Completing the module successfully will normally provide some form of certificate of achievement or a number of academic credits.

Numeracy: the ability to work with information that is in the form of numbers.

NVQ: National Vocational Qualifications are UK-based qualifications that are generally obtainable by adults through learning in the workplace. They are based on the demonstration of particular competencies.

OSCE: Objective Structured Clinical Examination – a formal and highly structured method of assessing practical skills.

Outline: a brief description, this term is sometimes used in relation to learning outcomes and written assessments.

Peer assessment: feedback from others in your group or other students whom you work with in placement.

Peers: those who are your equals, such as other students in your group.

Personal development plan: a written document that identifies a person's future learning needs, short- and long-term development goals and how these will be achieved.

Personal tutor: a named member of the academic staff who will provide academic support and guidance as well as a degree of pastoral care.

Placement: any area of health care or nursing practice where nursing or midwifery students may be allocated for a learning experience.

Plagiarism: using another person's ideas and passing them off as your own.

Policy: guide stating standard required responses to a situation; may be national (e.g. from the Department of Health) or local (e.g. from a Trust).

Portfolio: a collection of certificates, qualifications and testimonials, records of achievements and examples of work which demonstrates a learner's knowledge, skills and attitudes, and shows progression over a period of time.

Poster: a large sheet of paper that attempts to catch the eye and to communicate information on a topic. Sometime used as a form of assessment.

Practice educator: an individual who helps students to learn in the practice situation. Often serves as a link between mentors and their students. Different terms are used in different training localities.

Psychomotor skill: a skill that requires the coordination of mind and muscles.

Reference (for a job): prospective employers may refer to someone who knows you or has employed you for an evaluation of your past performance to determine your suitability for a job.

Reference to literature: this phrase will be used by your tutors and may be stated, as criteria, in assignments. This means that you should explicitly refer to published work by using direct quotes or by paraphrasing an author's idea in your essay. This would not include your class notes from a lecture.

Reflection: a focused retrospective activity which explores an issue of concern or interest through which learning and greater understanding of events is achieved.

Self-directed study: university students are expected to organise and undertake study on their own and in groups to supplement the classroom sessions taught by lecturers. Guidance on the amount of self-directed study which should be undertaken can be obtained from course or personal tutors.

Seminar: a small group of students (usually 10–20) discussing an issue under the direction of a teacher; often one person will lead. Less formal than a lecture.

Study plan or timetable: students should formulate a plan of their self-directed study each week/month.

Summative assignment: this is usually at the end of a course or module to determine if suffi-cient learning has taken place to award a pass grade and to provide feedback in a formally recorded mark.

Textbook: a book intended for study or instruction.

Time management: the art of getting things done that need to be done in the time available.

Timetable: in education this means the dates, times, titles, speakers and duration of planned sessions.

Transferable skill: a skill or ability that is useful in a wide number of professions or circumstances.

Tutor: academic member of staff who will advise and help you with your studies on a one-to-one basis.

Tutorial: refers to a small group of students (usually about five) discussing an issue. It can also refer to discussing an academic or practice issue with your tutor on a one-to-one basis.

Viva: short for viva voce, an oral examination.

White Paper: UK government report requiring mandatory actions.

Workbook: a book devised to stimulate learning by providing a series of activities and tasks that require completing.

Workshop: similar to a seminar although the learning is often driven through participation in a series of activities designed to stimulate thinking or to provide an opportunity to practise.

References

Annis, L. and Davis, J. K. (1978) Study techniques and cognitive styles: their effect on recall and recognition. *Journal of Educational Research*, 71: 175–178.

Arnold, G. (1998) Refinements in the dimensional analysis of dose calculation problem-solving. *Nurse Educator*, 23(3): 22–26

Astin, A. W. (1993) *What matters in college? Four critical years revisited*. San Francisco: Jossey-Bass.

Baly, M. ed (1991) As Miss Nightingale said . . . London: Scutari Press.

Beard, R. (1990) *Developing reading*. 2nd ed. London: Hodder and Stoughton.

Bloom, B. (1956) *Taxonomy of educational objectives*. New York: David McKay.

Brookfield, S. (1986) *Understanding and facilitating adult learning*. Buckingham: Open University Press.

Brown, G. and Atkins, M. (1988) *Effective teaching in higher education*. London: Methuen.

Bulman, C. and Schutz, S. (2004) *Reflective practice in nursing*. 3rd ed. Oxford: Blackwell.

Chandler, S. (2004) *100 ways to motivate yourself: change your life forever*. New Jersey: Career Press.

Chisholm, J. (2004) *Improve your spelling*. London: Usborne.

Clarke, C. (1999) *More grub on less grant: the new student cookbook*. London: Headline.

Conan Doyle, A. (1892) *The adventure of the beryl coronet*. London: Strand Magazine (May).

DeFina, A. A. (1992) *Portfolio assessment: getting started*. New York: Scholastic Professional Books.

Dunn, R. and Dunn K. (1978) *Teaching students through their learning styles: a practical approach*. Reston, VA: Reston Publishing

Dunn, R., Griggs, S., Olson, J., Beasley, M. and Gorman, B. (1995) A meta-analytical validation of the Dunn and Dunn model of learning style preferences. *Journal of Educational Research*, 88(6): 353–362.

Ebbinghaus, H. (1885) *Memory: a contribution to experimental psychology*. New York: Teachers College, Columbia University.

Entwistle, N. (1997) *Styles of learning and teaching: an integrated outline of educational psychology for students, teachers and lecturers*. London: David Fulton.

Fairbairn, G. J. and Winch, C. (1996) *Reading, writing and reasoning: a guide for students*. 2nd ed. Buckingham: Open University Press.

Felder, R. M. (1993) Reaching the second tier: learning and teaching styles in college education. *Journal of College Science Teaching*, 23: 286–290.

Fitts, P. M. and Posner, M. I. (1967) *Human performance*. Belmont, CA: Brooks/Cole.

Frank, A. R., Wacker, D. P., Keith, T. Z. and Sagen, T. K. (1987) Effectiveness of a spelling study package for learning disabled students. *Learning Disabilities Research*, 2: 110–118.

Fry, H., Ketteridge, S. and Marshall, S. (1999) *A handbook for teaching and learning in higher education: enhancing academic practice*. London: Kogan Page.

Gardner, H. (1993) *Frames of mind: the theory of multiple intelligences*. 10th ed. New York: Basic Books.

Gibbs, G. (1988) *Learning by doing: a guide to teaching and learning methods*. Oxford: Further Education Unit, Oxford Polytechnic.

Greene, H. A. (1954) *The new Iowa spelling scale*. Iowa City: University of Iowa.

Hadley, J. C. (1999) I can't. *Journal of PeriAnesthesia Nursing*, 14(3): 160–162.

Harden, R. M. and Gleeson, F. A. (1979) Assessment of clinical competence using objective structured clinical examinations (OSCE). *Medical Education*, 13: 41–54.

Hill, W. (1985) *Learning: a survey of psychological interpretations*. 4th ed. New York: Harper and Row.

Honey, P. and Mumford, A. (1992) *The manual of learning styles*. 3rd ed. Maidenhead: Peter Honey.

Howell, W. C. and Fleishman, E. A. eds. (1982) Human performance and productivity. Vol 2: *Information processing and decision making*. Hillsdale, NJ: Erlbaum.

Hull, C., Redfern, L. and Shuttleworth, A. (2005) *Profiles and portfolios: a guide for health and social care*. 2nd ed. Basingstoke: Palgrave.

Irving, N. (2004a) *Improve your grammar*. London: Usborne.

Irving, N. (2004b) *Improve your punctuation*. London: Usborne.

Jasper, M. A. (1999) Nurses' perceptions of the value of written reflection. *Nurse Education Today*, 19: 452–463.

Jenkins, A. (1998) *Curriculum design in geography*. Cheltenham: Geography Discipline Network, Cheltenham and Gloucester College of Higher Education.

Johns, C. (1992) The Burford Nursing Development Unit holistic model of nursing practice. *Journal of Advanced Nursing*, 16(10): 1090–1098 (Adapted).

Kesselman-Turkel, J. and Peterson, F. (1982) *Note-taking made easy*. Lincolnwood, IL: Contemporary Books.

Kiewra, K. A. (1987) Learning from a lecture: an investigation into note taking, review and attendance at a lecture. *Human Learning*, 4: 73–77.

Kiewra, K. A. and Benton, S. L. (1988) The relationship between information-processing ability and notetaking. *Contemporary Educational Psychology*, 13: 34–44.

Knaus, W. J. (1997) *Do it now: break the procrastination habit*. New York: Wiley.

Knowles, M. S. (1986) *Using learning contracts*. San Francisco, CA: Jossey-Bass.

Kolb, D. A. (1984) *Experiential learning: experience as the source of learning and development*. Englewood Cliffs, NJ: Prentice Hall.

Kulhavy, R. W. and Dyer, J. W. (1975) The effects of notetaking and test expectancy on the learning of text material. *Journal of Educational Research*, 68: 363–365.

Lapham, R. and Agar, H. (2003) *Drug calculations for nurses: a step-by-step approach*. 2nd ed. London: Arnold.

Lawler, G. (2003) *Understanding maths: basic mathematics for adults explained*. Abergele: Studymates.

Liebman, B. (2002) Face the fats. *Nutrition Action Newsletter*, July/August: 3–6.

Mason D. J. and Kohn, M. L. (2001) *The memory workbook: breakthrough techniques to exercise your memory*. London: New Harbinger Books.

Newton, D. and Smith, D. (2003) *Practice in basic skills: maths*. London: HarperCollins.

Nicol, M., Bavin, C., Bedford-Turner, S., Cronin, P. and Rawlings-Anderson, K. (2004) *Essential nursing skills*. 2nd ed. Edinburgh: Mosby.

Nursing and Midwifery Council (2002a) *An NMC guide for students of nursing and midwifery*. London: NMC.

Nursing and Midwifery Council (2002b) *Guidelines for records and record keeping*. London: NMC.

Nursing and Midwifery Council (2004) *The NMC Code of professional conduct: standards for conduct, performance and ethics*. London: NMC.

O'Brien, D. (2003) *Never forget facts and figures*. London: Duncan Baird.

O'Brien, E. T., Petrie, J. C., Littler, W. A. et al (1997) *Blood pressure measurement: recommendations of the British Hypertension Society*. 3rd ed. London: British Medical Journal.

Oermann, M. H. and Ziolkowski, L. D. (2002) Accuracy of references in three critical care nursing journals. *Journal of PeriAnesthesia Nursing*, 17(2): 78–83.

Pascarella, E. T. and Terenzini, P. T. (1991) *How college affects students: findings and insights from twenty years of research*. San Francisco: Jossey-Bass.

Pauk, W. (1993) *How to study in college*. Boston, MA: Houghton Mifflin.

Payne, E. and Whittaker, L. (2000) *Developing essential study skills*. London: Pearson.

Pearson, A., Vaughan, B. and FitzGerald, M. (2005) *Nursing models in practice*. 3rd ed. Oxford: Elsevier Science.

Powell, S. (1999) *Returning to study: a guide for professionals*. Buckingham: Open University Press.

Quinn, F. M. (2000) *Principles and practice of nurse education*. 4th ed. Cheltenham: Stanley Thornes.

Ramsden, P. (1992) *Learning to teach in higher education*. London: Routledge.

Riding, R. and Rayner, S. (1998) *Cognitive styles and learning strategies: understanding style differences in learning and behaviour*. London: David Fulton.

Robinson, P. (1961) *Effective study*. New York: Harper and Row.

Rogers, J. (1989) *Adults learning*. 3rd ed. Milton Keynes: Open University Press.

Rolfe, G., Freshwater, D. and Jasper, M. (2001) *Critical reflection for nursing*. Basingstoke: Palgrave.

Rose, J. (2001) *The mature student's guide to writing*. Basingstoke: Palgrave.

Rowntree, D. (1998) *Learn how to study: a realistic approach*. 4th ed. London: Time Warner.

Schon, D. (1999) *The reflective practitioner: how professionals think in action*. London: Ashgate.

Sinclair, A. and Wesinger, R. (2004) Omega-3 fatty acids and the brain. *Chemistry in Australia*, Nov: 6–10.

Smith, A. (2001) *Accelerated learning in practice*. Stafford: Network Educational Press.

Straker, A. (1995–1996) *Mental maths*. Vols 1–6. Cambridge: Cambridge University Press.

Sully, P. and Dallas, J. (2005) *Essential communication skills for nursing*. Edinburgh: Mosby.

Tapper, J. (2004) Student perceptions of how critical thinking is embedded in a degree program. *Higher Education Research and Development*, 23(2): 199–222.

Truss, L. (2003) *Eats, shoots and leaves: the zero tolerance approach to punctuation*. London: Profile Books.

Usher, K., Francis, D. and Owens, J. (1999) Reflective writing: a strategy to foster critical inquiry in undergraduate nursing students. *Australian Journal of Advanced Nursing*, 17(1): 7–12.

VanDyck, W. (1996) *Punctuation repair kit*. London: Hodder Children's Books.

Williams, S. (2005) Head games: the use of mental rehearsal to improve performance. Online. Available: www.wright.edu/~scott.williams/LeaderLetter/rehearsal.htm.

Wright, J. (2002) Time management: the pickle jar theory. *A List Apart*, 146. Online. Available: www.alistapart.com/articles/pickle.

Index